FODMAP
FRIENDLY

FODMAP Friendly: *95 Vegetarian & Gluten-Free Recipes for the Digestively Challenged*
Text and photographs copyright © 2018, 2020 by Georgia McDermott
Photographs on pages 16–17 (top), 88–89 (left), 124–125, 150–151, 178–179, and 215, and
author photograph copyright © 2018, 2020 by Elisa Watson

Originally published in Australia by Pan Macmillan Australia Pty Ltd in 2018. First published
in North America in revised form by The Experiment, LLC, in 2020.

The Experiment, LLC | 220 East 23rd Street, Suite 600 | New York, NY 10010-4658
theexperimentpublishing.com

This book contains the opinions and ideas of its author. It is intended to provide helpful and
informative material on the subjects addressed in the book. It is sold with the understanding
that the author and publisher are not engaged in rendering medical, health, or any other kind
of personal professional services in the book. The author and publisher specifically disclaim
all responsibility for any liability, loss, or risk—personal or otherwise—that is incurred as a
consequence, directly or indirectly, of the use and application of any of the contents of this book.

THE EXPERIMENT and its colophon are registered trademarks of The Experiment, LLC. Many
of the designations used by manufacturers and sellers to distinguish their products are claimed
as trademarks. Where those designations appear in this book and The Experiment was aware
of a trademark claim, the designations have been capitalized.

The Experiment's books are available at special discounts when purchased in bulk for
premiums and sales promotions as well as for fund-raising or educational use. For details,
contact us at info@theexperimentpublishing.com.

Library of Congress Cataloging-in-Publication Data

Names: McDermott, Georgia, author.
Title: Fodmap friendly : 95 vegetarian & gluten-free recipes for the
    digestively challenged / Georgia McDermott.
Description: New York : The Experiment, 2020. | Includes index.
Identifiers: LCCN 2020024433 (print) | LCCN 2020024434 (ebook) | ISBN
    9781615197040 (trade paperback) | ISBN 9781615197057 (ebook)
Subjects: LCSH: Vegetarian cooking. | Gluten-free diet--Recipes.
Classification: LCC TX837 .M4754 2020 (print) | LCC TX837 (ebook) | DDC
    641.5/636--dc23
LC record available at https://lccn.loc.gov/2020024433
LC ebook record available at https://lccn.loc.gov/2020024434

ISBN 978-1-61519-704-0
Ebook ISBN 978-1-61519-705-7

Cover design by Jack Dunnington
Text design by Arielle Gamble

Manufactured in China

First printing September 2020
10 9 8 7 6 5 4 3 2 1

FODMAP FRIENDLY

95 VEGETARIAN & GLUTEN-FREE Recipes
for the Digestively Challenged

GEORGIA McDERMOTT

THE EXPERIMENT

NEW YORK

Contents

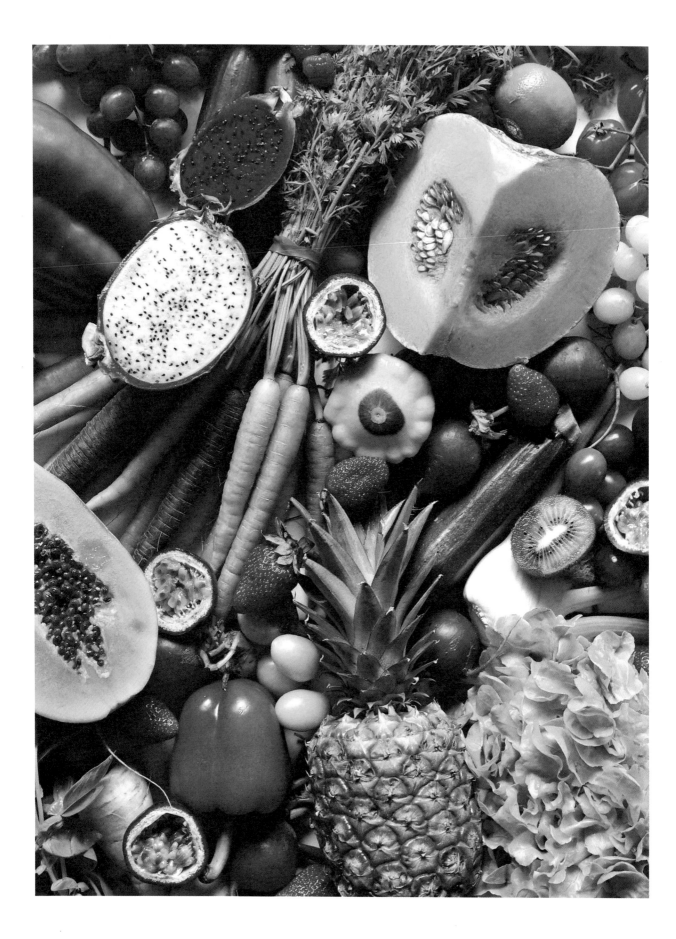

Introduction

My relationship with food? It's complicated . . .

They say the ones you love hurt you the most, and this is definitely true of my relationship with food. My fierce love of food is paralleled only by my body's fierce rejection of practically everything I eat. This tumultuous relationship has been a theme throughout my life, starting with minor discomforts and progressively worsening to the current day, where I can bloat up and be out of action in a matter of hours. *Guinness World Records*, are you listening?

The fact that my love of food was unrequited was apparent even when I was a tiny human. I'd complain of a hot tummy constantly, and randomly reject foods like pasta or bread. My first experience with elimination diets (unbeknownst to me at the time) was at age ten with the candida diet—from that, I learned never to trust Mum again (or at least never to let her buy untoasted almond butter).

These food-related niggles continued on through school. I'd feel nauseated by foods that I'd enjoyed the week before, much to Mum's frustration. Given that they were just niggles, I didn't pay too much attention—that is, until I reached university, when it became apparent that I was more than just a fussy eater. Throughout my second year, I had a constant, throbbing headache behind one eye,

and the nausea became more commonplace. CT scans and visits to doctors failed to diagnose my ill health, so, as every good millennial does, I took charge of my own destiny and began researching on the internet. What I came up with was the idea to change my diet and go gluten-free. I took this to my doctor, who was pretty disinclined to believe that food could be making me sick—instead, she suggested that I stop studying in bed and invest in a desk. Frustrated that nobody understood my condition or seemed to take me seriously, I set about cleaning up my diet and going gluten-free on my own. Was it a magic bullet? Yes and no. For a while, the headaches dissipated, the nausea subsided, and I felt like I could function again. To carry on the theme of cheesy clichés, however, all good things must come to an end, and so it was with my newfound magic cure. Suddenly and without warning I was constantly bloated, nauseous, full, and exhausted, and, to put it mildly, my digestive system had gone wild.

The next year or two were characterized by more visits to doctors' offices and tests—endoscopies, colonoscopies, nuclear medicine tests, blood tests, stool tests, whatever tests. From the nuclear medicine exam, I was diagnosed on the spot with gastroparesis, a condition where the nerves responsible for the muscle contractions that push food through the digestive system are damaged or not functioning as they should. It can be caused by physical injury, a virus, or diabetes, or it can be idiopathic (i.e., your doctor has no idea what caused it), as mine was. Gastroparesis manifests in the form of exceedingly slow digestion, feeling full and bloated, nutritional deficiencies, and, often, imbalances in your intestinal flora. I'm lucky that my case was relatively mild—some people are unable to keep food down at all and have to be fed via a tube.

When adhering to the guidelines for this condition failed to improve the symptoms, I searched for other solutions. I noticed that most doctors I encountered during this time were reluctant to believe that food might be causing my ill health. They searched for external factors, such as stress—one gastroenterologist even suggested that walking around on concrete floors had made my organs "saggy"—but none turned to food and nutrition as a factor. Considering food is a common denominator in every single day, I found this hard to stomach. (Gastroparesis puns! Fun!)

Finally, a light at the end of the tunnel

On the advice of a friend, I made an appointment with an integrative doctor. An integrative doctor, before you slam this book shut, is a qualified medical doctor who incorporates a holistic, nutrition-focused approach to their practice. This particular doctor's interest in diet and the role that it plays in digestive illness (a shocking idea, really) was the catalyst in my decision to try a new path of healing. After all, I couldn't avoid concrete floors for the rest of my life.

Pretty quickly, my integrative doctor (and new hero) diagnosed me with SIBO, or small intestinal bacterial overgrowth. As its name suggests, SIBO is the over-colonization of bacteria in the small intestine, an area of the digestive system where these bacteria are not supposed to reside. This imbalance results in bloating, gas, nausea, altered bowel movements, and, among other things, (wait for it) food intolerances.

My two illnesses had a symbiotic relationship. My slow-moving digestion provided the ultimate feeding ground for the bacteria that had overgrown there, and, in turn, the unwanted overgrowth of bacteria was slowing down my peristaltic wave (the muscle contraction that pushes food through). It was a fun, fun time.

If you're reading this book, chances are you probably know at least a little bit about FODMAPs. In absolute layman's terms, FODMAPs are short-chain carbohydrates (sugars and related molecules) found naturally in many foods, or added to them. Unlike other sugars, they aren't absorbed in the small intestine. Foods high in FODMAPs carry on down to the large intestine, where they are easily fermented by bacteria, causing gas, bloating, and a whole host of other (un)pleasant symptoms.

The FODMAP acronym breaks down like this:
Fermentable (used as a food source by the bacteria in the large intestine)
Oligosaccharides (a chain of individual sugars)
Disaccharides (a double sugar known as lactose)
Monosaccharides (excess fructose)
And
Polyols (sugar alcohols such as sorbitol, mannitol, and xylitol).

Some of the most common FODMAP offenders are onion, garlic, lactose, fructose, and wheat.

Enter FODMAPs

So, what happened next? I tried the whole spectrum of relevant antibiotics, desperately clinging to the newfound light at the end of the tunnel. After each failure, I'd return to my doctor, and we'd discuss the next one to try. During this trial and error process (a side effect of which included virtually wiping out my intestinal flora), I was given an intermediary option: the low-FODMAP diet. I'd encountered this intimidating acronym when I was "doctor googling" my headaches, but, back then, I had failed to read past the first few sentences of science-laden text. (Always was, always will be, an arts student.)

In the early days, I had felt that my symptoms didn't warrant the removal of so many foods from my diet. This time, however, it was basically a matter of eliminating a few dispensable and niche items—such was the state of my worsening intolerances. This is how I unglamorously and unceremoniously started the low-FODMAP diet.

At this point, it would tie up nice and neatly if I said that the low-FODMAP diet was the magic bullet that cured me, but nothing in my life is neat—not my wardrobe, not my hair, and certainly not my digestive health. I know it's trendy to write a book after the fact, to emerge from ill health having "cured yourself" and promising to do the same for others. But I haven't cured myself. I'm still sick, near daily, and it impacts most aspects of my life, from socializing, to dating, to what I wear (criteria: it must float to hide the bloat).

As a result of these as-yet uncured illnesses and intolerances, every meal I eat is a highly considered decision. I have to factor in what it consists of, whether the portion size will make me sick, how long it has been since my last meal, and whether or not I'm willing to throw caution to the wind and potentially feel sick for the next few days. The hardest part about a digestive illness is that people see you out eating pizza, but they don't see, or feel, what happens to you afterward. So, I'm not healed, but what the low-FODMAP diet *has* given me is a framework around which to base my food choices.

Given the nature of my work (cooking and testing food on a near-daily basis), it has proven impossible to follow a dietary protocol to the letter. However, armed with knowledge from the creators of the low-FODMAP diet (and particularly Dr. Sue Shepherd, who has written a number of books on the subject), I am able to make the smartest choices possible in terms of what I eat (I'm open to suggestions for smart choices in other aspects of my life, though!). There are plenty of resources out there to guide you through your digestive difficulties, and I would always recommend starting with your primary care physician or health practitioner.

So, yes, the ones you love might hurt you the most, but they might also present you with opportunities that you never dreamed of (surely the title of a novella or an Instagram poem somewhere?). A situation I thought was wildly unfair ultimately gave me the things I am most passionate about and proud of: my career in food and this cookbook.

Going Public

When a mishap during a routine wisdom tooth removal laid me up in bed for a month, I decided I needed a hobby to occupy my newfound free time. I'd recently downloaded

Instagram and, at the behest of my twenty-odd followers, had taken to uploading my sloppy attempts at poached eggs. As my "likes" dwindled, I decided that my friends were an ungrateful and unappreciative audience, and I created a secret Instagram account called @georgeats.

Just as Zuckerberg intended, I became consumed with the likes and the comments. More than that, though, I began interacting with, and being inspired by, fellow food Instagrammers. I learnt a lot about gluten-free alternatives from strangers and hashtags, which was a new concept. It's hard to believe with all the smoothie-bowl accounts these days, but at the time it was a relatively small community.

Once I finished university and started working part-time, I dedicated all my spare time to photographing food and posting on Insta, using the wages from my two jobs to fund my excessive gluten-free-flour usage, and my days off to play around with my entry-level camera and two ceramic plates. My boss introduced me to a PR company who offered me an ongoing freelance job in social media content creation. This opportunity was the first of many catalysts that pushed my unorthodox career in the direction it has gone, at the speed that it has.

As my photography improved, I started a blog. Still searching for answers to my digestive issues, the blog became an outlet to post my gluten-free and FODMAP-friendly recipes, and to occasionally send a frustrated whine about my health out into the ether. Both the blog and my Insta account have grown exponentially since then, inspiring me to write this cookbook.

I hope this book will be helpful for people who are struggling with digestive issues, who are new to FODMAPs, or who still believe that a bill of (better) health isn't worth having to lose entire food groups and flavors from their diets. I've been all three of those people.

Use the book to explore what does and doesn't work for you. Digestive systems are extremely personal, and everyone has a nuanced reaction to food. For example, I don't tolerate many grains (FODMAP friendly or not), so I only eat them occasionally. Onion and garlic don't bother you? Add them! The thought of tomatoes makes you nauseous? Don't eat them! Remember, the whole point is to feel better. If something doesn't sit well with you, acknowledge it, work around it, and substitute with other foods. This book will hopefully provide you with ideas and inspiration to experiment with a way of eating that suits you.

A note on meat: I am a pescatarian for both ethical reasons and taste preferences, but meat is very much FODMAP friendly. If you'd like to incorporate meat into any of these dishes, do so freely, but use your own cooking smarts. I can't give you any directions—I haven't cooked meat in ten years, and my mentality when I did so was to "cook it until it's burnt to make sure there's nothing raw about it." Might this have something to do with my displeasure at the taste? I guess we'll never know.

The No-Go Zone

Here is a hit list of the most common high-FODMAP foods (though some only fall into this category above certain amounts).

Remember, everyone is different, and you may not have a problem with some of these foods—it's a matter of trial and error. If you find that you have no issues with an ingredient listed, don't exclude it for no reason.

This is by no means an exhaustive list: There's lots more information available online, including complete lists of high-FODMAP foods and the quantities in which they become a problem. Most of the foods on this list have an acceptable threshold for consumption. You might even see some of them in my recipes! The point of the low-FODMAP diet is to minimize inclusion of foods that can cause digestive distress, while still maintaining a varied diet.

I use the Monash University Low FODMAP Diet Guide app to help me work out the FODMAP content of specific foods. All the information I've provided in this book on the FODMAP content of foods is correct at time of printing; but testing methods are improving all the time, which can slightly alter a food's FODMAP levels.

Fruits

- Apples
- Apricots
- Blackberries
- Cherries
- Dried fruit
- Fruit juice
- Mangoes
- Nectarines
- Peaches
- Pears
- Plums
- Pomegranates
- Watermelon

Vegetables

- Artichokes
- Asparagus
- Beets
- Butternut squash
- Cauliflower
- Celery
- Garlic
- Green peas
- Leeks
- Mushrooms
- Onions
- Scallions (white part only)
- Shallots
- Sugar snap peas
- Sweet corn

Milk and milk products

- Cow's milk, goat's milk, soy milk
- Custard
- Ice cream
- Soft cheeses: cottage cheese, ricotta, quark, cream cheese, mascarpone, crème fraîche
- Yogurt

Other foods

- Barley-, rye-, and wheat-based commercial bread, bread crumbs, breakfast cereals, muesli, pasta, couscous, gnocchi, noodles, pastries, cakes, biscuits, croissants, muffins
- Flours (in large amounts), including chickpea flour (besan), lentil flour, pea flour, soy flour
- Rye (in large amounts)
- Wheat (in large amounts), including bulgur, durum, wheat flour, multigrain flour, triticale, wheat germ, wheat bran, semolina
- Wheat-based crackers, crispbreads
- Almonds; cashews; hazelnuts; pistachios
- Chickpeas
- Hummus
- Tahini
- Legumes
- Lentils
- Honey

My Low-FODMAP Pantry

Flours and Other Baking Staples

I use a variety of flours for my cooking, some of which may be unfamiliar to you if you haven't had to delve into these dark arts before. That said, they are all easily acquired at supermarkets (check both the baking and health aisles, or pester a clerk if you're completely lost), health food stores, or bulk food stores. Most of these products are relatively inexpensive, and best of all by using them you will have full control over what's in your baked goods.

Personally, I'm not a fan of pre-mixed flour blends, as each contains a wildly different mix of flours, inevitably affecting the end result. More than that, a lot of them contain gums, which assist in binding, but often to the detriment of digestive comfort. Some even contain beans!

Almond meal

Almond meal is considered a "safe" food in amounts up to ¼ cup, so the recipes included in this book reflect that. It lends a beautiful, nutty crumb to baked goods and is great for those who need to avoid grains.

Baking powder (gluten-free)

Not all baking powders are created equal, so make sure the one you choose is gluten-free, particularly if you are baking for a celiac.

Buckwheat flour

Buckwheat is actually a gluten-free seed, bearing no relation to FODMAP-unfriendly wheat. It lends a very distinct nutty flavor to baking and soaks up liquid like nobody's business, so it's best used in smaller amounts and in conjunction with other flours.

Millet flour

Millet flour is a nutty, sweet, yet bitter flour made from the milled millet grain. It adds a nice taste and texture to baked goods, but use it only in smaller quantities to keep bitterness at a minimum.

Oat flour

I make my own oat flour by grinding gluten-free rolled oats in my food processor. Oats are FODMAP friendly in amounts up to ½ cup, even if they aren't gluten-free oats. I use gluten-free because of my personal dietary concerns, but if you don't strictly need to be gluten-free, you can use regular oats.

Potato starch

Potato starch has a light consistency, similar to tapioca flour or cornstarch, and is great for holding moisture in baked goods (like the Pizza Crusts on page 189).

Psyllium husk

This magic ingredient shows up in a few of my baking recipes. Psyllium husk is a natural, inexpensive, and slightly frightening ingredient that gels up on contact with liquid, mimicking the elasticity of traditional dough. (Xanthan and guar gum perform a similar job, so I've heard, but they're known for causing digestive distress, which is why I've never used them.)

Quinoa flour

A sweet, nutty-flavored option, quinoa flour adds a nice flavor and texture to baked goods. It is also quite high in protein.

Rice flour (white and brown)

Rice flours often form the bulk of gluten-free flour blends and gluten-free baked goods in general. They are inexpensive, easy to find, and easy to use. Make sure you get a finely ground variety—coarse rice flour will leave you with a gritty texture. I find there's a subtle difference between each flour, although some people use them interchangeably.

Tapioca flour

I use tapioca flour in basically everything I bake—it complements all the other flours listed here. On its own, it becomes a gummy, chewy mess, so be sure to use it as a way to lighten up dense flours, rather than by itself. It is similar to cornstarch in its ability to thicken sauces, but as corn is a common food intolerance, I prefer tapioca.

Sugars

There's a world of sugar substitutes out there, but the FODMAP-friendliest varieties, somewhat ironically in the current climate of wellness, are the refined sort. Whichever variety you choose, consuming sugar in superhuman amounts is a recipe for an unhappy digestive system. Something to bear in mind when you're on your fourth macaron.

Brown sugar

Brown sugar is my favorite FODMAP-friendly sweetener, as it lends a great caramelly depth of flavor to baked goods. Here, I've used light brown sugar—the darker the sugar gets, the more molasses it contains (a FODMAP-unfriendly sweetener), so keep that in mind when experimenting with dark brown sugar.

Coconut sugar

While coconut sugar is touted as a "healthy" alternative to regular sugar, it's actually quite high in fructose and therefore not always suitable for use in FODMAP-friendly baking, particularly in large quantities. Servings in excess of 4 teaspoons are considered high in both fructose and oligos, so while I do use some coconut sugar, I keep the serving size well under this amount.

Maple syrup

A low-FODMAP serving is 2½ tablespoons of maple syrup. It's a good substitute for honey in terms of consistency, but make sure you are buying pure, unadulterated maple syrup—there are loads of maple syrup–flavored sweeteners on the market, which contain a whole cocktail of different sugar sources.

Brown rice syrup

Brown rice syrup is a low-FODMAP sweetener with the consistency of thick honey, which makes it good for holding things together (like my Granola Bars on page 126). Be aware that some rice syrups are made with barley extract and are therefore not gluten-free. This doesn't present an issue for the FODMAP diet, but it does if you are celiac.

White sugar and confectioners' sugar
Having unlearned everything I learned in my early cooking days about refined-sugar-free ingredients being infinitely better for you (spoiler alert: in FODMAP terms, sugar is sugar), I now use a moderate amount of white sugar in my baking, as and when necessary. White, superfine (caster), and confectioners' sugars are all FODMAP friendly, so you can use them freely (within reason).

Fats and Oils

Fats and oils are FODMAP friendly. Some people can be sensitive to foods with a high fat content, but as a general rule, the below all have the green light:

- Butter
- Coconut oil
- Plant-based butter
- Olive oil and extra virgin olive oil
- Other nut and seed oils

Flavorings

You might think all is lost in the absence of onion and garlic, but fear not. Add a few (or all, if you're really daring) of these as a way to jazz up an otherwise basic meal.

- Apple cider vinegar
- Capers and caper berries
- Furikake (A dry Japanese seasoning you can sprinkle over all types of things, it contains chopped seaweed, sesame seeds, dried fish flakes, salt, and sugar; I make my own, without the dried fish flakes—see page 119.)
- Galangal, ginger, and lemongrass
- Herbs and spices, fresh or dried

- Homemade stock (There's a recipe for a veggie one on page 62.)
- Hot sauce (Make sure it doesn't contain onion or garlic; Tabasco is a good option.)
- Makrut lime leaves and makrut limes (more about these on page 63)
- *Kecap manis* (Indonesian sweet soy sauce)
- Lemons and limes
- Miso paste
- Mustard
- Nori
- Pickles
- Preserved lemon
- Tamari (A soy sauce with little or no wheat, tamari is not always gluten-free, so check the label to make sure.)

Fruits

Excess fructose can be a trigger for a lot of people, so stick to these fruits if it's a concern for you.

- Acai (puree packets and powder)
- Bananas
- Blueberries, raspberries, and strawberries
- Cantaloupe
- Citrus fruits
- Dragonfruit
- Grapes
- Guava
- Kiwifruits
- Papaya
- Passion fruit
- Pineapple
- Rhubarb

Vegetables

Veggies are a low-FODMAPper's best friend. There are plenty of vegetables you can eat with reckless abandon, to bulk up both your general diet and fiber intake.

- Beets (Canned beet is friendly in ½-cup servings.)
- Bell peppers
- Bok choy and Asian greens
- Broccoli (friendly in 1-cup servings)
- Cabbage (but avoid savoy)
- Carrots
- Celeriac
- Chile peppers
- Cucumbers
- Edamame
- Eggplant
- Fennel (friendly up to ½-cup servings)
- Greens (spinach, kale, chard, etc.)
- Green beans (friendly in small servings, 12 beans or fewer)
- Lettuce
- Olives
- Parsnips
- Potatoes
- Radishes
- Spinach
- Squash (Butternut is friendly only up to ¼-cup servings.)
- Tomatoes (Grape and cherry tomatoes are only low-FODMAP in varying degrees, but the regular variety are low-FODMAP.)

Dairy

I mean, who wants to live without cheese? A lot of cheese, despite popular opinion, is low enough in lactose to be FODMAP friendly. This is particularly relevant for hard cheeses like Parmesan, which have almost negligible amounts. (Something to note: Cheeses can often be made with an enzyme derived from animal rennet, so look for a vegetarian-friendly brand if you're vegetarian.) Use freshly, finely grated Parmesan from a wedge. Pre-grated Parmesan often contains fillers, which can be irritating to sensitive digestive systems.

Cheese
- Brie, Camembert
- Cheddar
- Cottage cheese
- Feta
- Goat cheese
- Halloumi (in two-slice servings)
- Mozzarella
- Parmesan, pecorino
- Swiss

Milk
- Lactose-free milk or cream (Though heavy cream is lower in lactose and friendly in small servings.)
- Lactose-free yogurt
- Coconut milk (Check that it doesn't contain inulin, a highly fermentable fiber found in things like leeks and asparagus. It's sometimes used as a thickener in coconut milk, and although it functions similarly to psyllium, it has a much higher tendency for malabsorption.)
- Rice milk
- Almond (or other nut) milk

Eggs

Eggs are indispensable! Unless otherwise specified, I use jumbo eggs in my baking recipes.

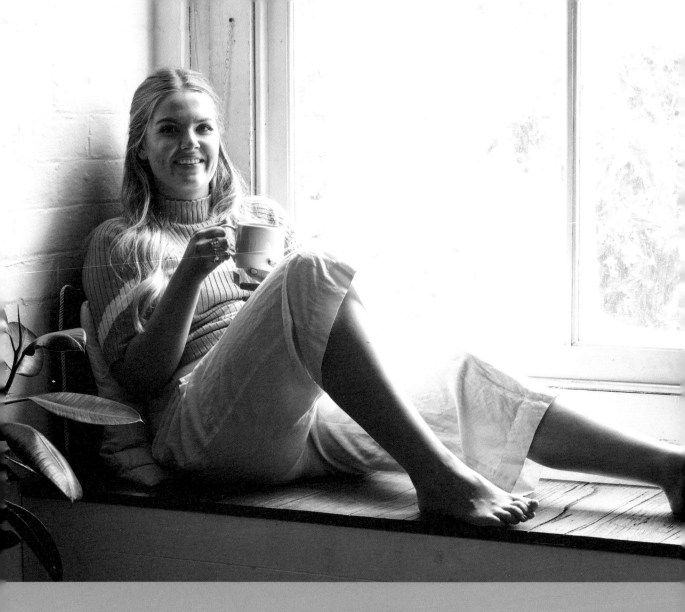

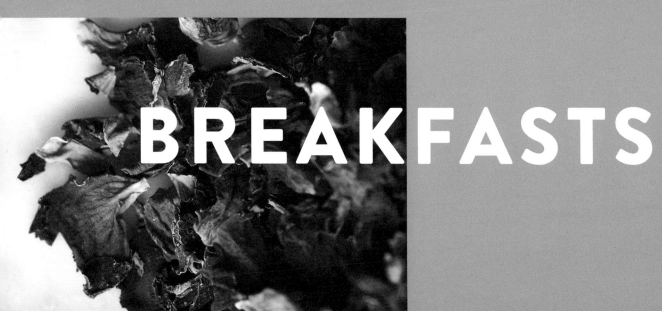

BREAKFASTS

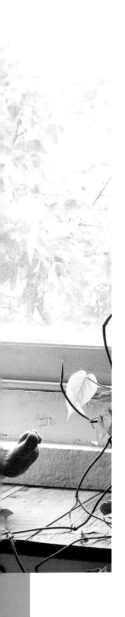

Some people's reason to wake up every morning is a pet or a significant other. Mine is breakfast. With a strong coffee and a mutual understanding that nobody in the house should try to interact with me until afterward, breakfast truly is the best time of the day.

.

For those who disagree: Have you ever woken up next to a bowl of choc-chip granola? It ain't half bad.

My choc-chip-granola boyfriend aside, I find that breakfast is the trickiest meal of the day to cater for. So many convenient foods are off the table, particularly if (as for me) store-bought gluten-free bread is not your friend.

As a result, I've filled this chapter with the whole gamut of breakfast foods—from quick and easy to weekend breakfast projects. Otherwise known as: plenty of things to wake up for (and no desert-dry bread).

Quinoa, Banana, and Blueberry Pancakes

MAKES 8
MEDIUM
PANCAKES

Why, yes (thanks for asking), I have spent considerable time deciding on my personal favorite pancake flavor . . . it's banana. That said, bananas do become increasingly FODMAP-unfriendly as they ripen, so consider using underripe bananas if you react badly to ripe ones.

2 ripe bananas
¾ cup (90 g) quinoa flour
½ cup (125 ml) almond milk
2 eggs, lightly beaten
1 tablespoon maple syrup
1 teaspoon vanilla bean paste or extract
1 teaspoon baking powder
1 teaspoon apple cider vinegar
½ cup (70 g) blueberries
Coconut oil or butter, for frying

To serve (optional)
Coconut yogurt or plain yogurt
Maple syrup
Blueberries
Grated dark chocolate

1. Mash the bananas thoroughly in a large bowl, and then add the quinoa flour, almond milk, and eggs. Stir well to combine, then add the maple syrup, vanilla, baking powder, and vinegar. If you don't mind losing the banana chunks, you can also do this in your food processor. Either way, once a batter has formed, gently stir in the blueberries.

2. Heat a nonstick frying pan over medium-low heat and melt a little coconut oil or butter in it.

3. Spoon about ¼ cup (60 ml) of the batter into the pan and allow it to cook for a few minutes, or until the top begins to bubble and the sides are solidifying. Gently flip the pancake over and cook for a few minutes on the other side. Transfer to a serving dish and cover to keep warm.

4. Repeat with the remaining batter, ensuring you grease the pan each time. Serve with the coconut yogurt, maple syrup, a few extra blueberries, and a bit (or a lot) of grated dark chocolate sprinkled on top, if desired.

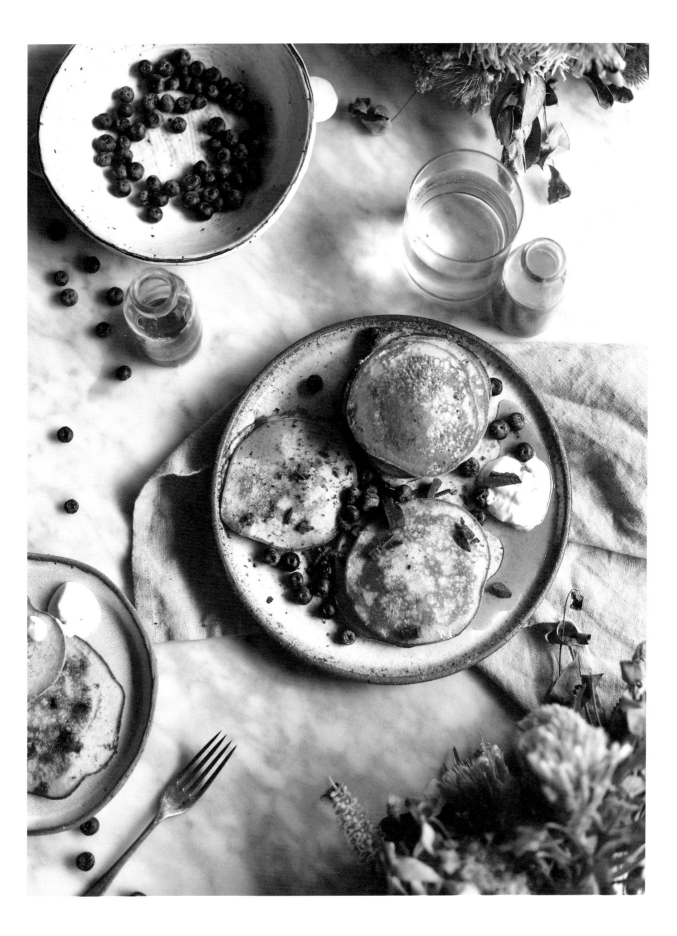

Acai Bowl, Two Ways

EACH BOWL SERVES 1

Hands up if you've ever been personally victimized by the amount of high-fructose fruit in coffee shop acai bowls? I've taken to making them at home—they're so easy and, much like my love life, there's not a single date in sight. I've included a frozen zucchini version for those who can't tolerate bananas and used powdered acai, because it's easy on the budget and is often easier to find. I've also designed the recipes so that you can add as few, or as many, of the optional extras as you like. Personally, I like blueberries, strawberries, coconut flakes, almonds, and seeds, like pumpkin, sunflower, and chia, on my bowls, although a rose petal or two doesn't go astray, if I'm snapping it for the 'gram—and often, I add them all.

Zucchini Bowl

1 small zucchini (100 g), sliced, steamed, cooled, and frozen the night before

2½ tablespoons peanut butter

1 tablespoon acai powder

2 teaspoons maple syrup or sweetener of your choice

2½ tablespoons almond milk or coconut cream

Toppings (optional)

2½ tablespoons protein powder

⅓ cup (50 g) frozen berries

¼ avocado, sliced

Banana Bowl

1 large banana, frozen (for lower fructose content, freeze bananas before they ripen)

1 cup (100 g) frozen berries (or frozen zucchini for a lower-fructose option)

1 tablespoon acai powder

1 tablespoon peanut butter

Toppings (optional)

2½ tablespoons protein powder

Handful of fresh berries

Coconut flakes

Flaked almonds

Pumpkin seeds

Sunflower seeds

Chia seeds

Poached rhubarb

1. Blend all the bowl ingredients together in a food processor until a thick, lump-free smoothie has formed. Adjust the liquid content and sweetness to your liking—I prefer a thick and barely sweet acai bowl.
2. Pour into a bowl and add the toppings of your choice.

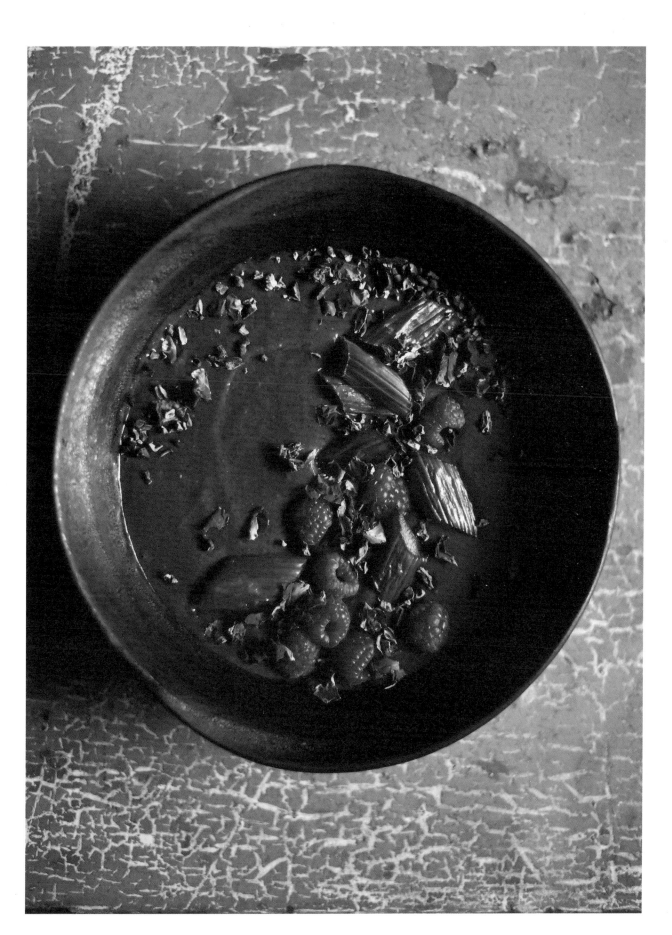

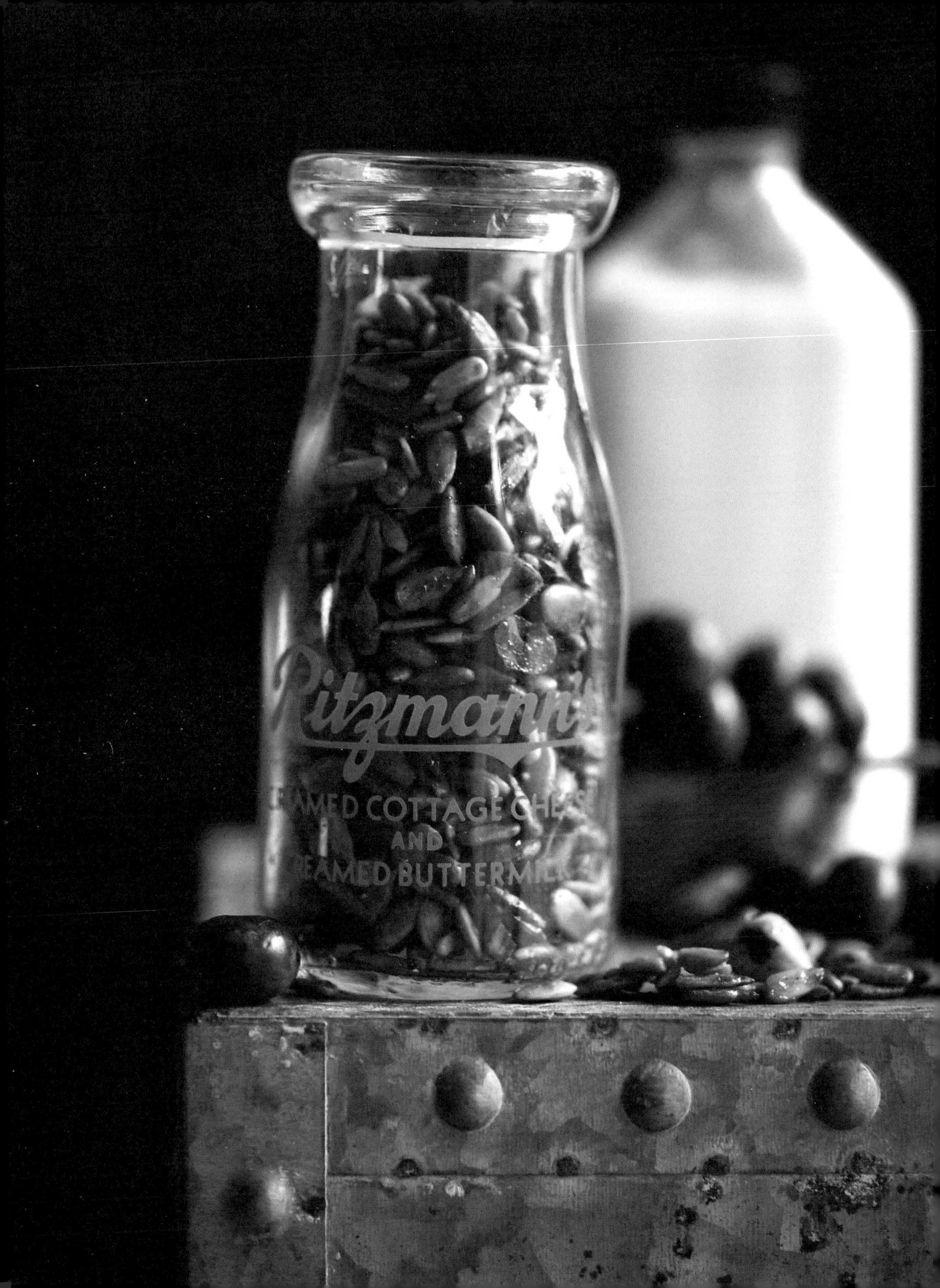
Ritzmann's
COTTAGE
AND

Grain-Free Olive Oil Granola

Does anyone else ever overcomplicate the process of making granola? I can't count the amount of times I've tried to remain relevant by coming up with an outrageously flavored granola concoction, only to end up with a clump of burnt nuts. Maybe people aren't lying when they say simple is best.

This granola is vegan, grain-free, and gluten-free and can also be made nut-free by swapping additional sunflower seeds and pepitas in place of the almonds and hazelnuts. Hot tip: The milk at the bottom of the bowl is arguably better than the granola itself.

2 cups (300 g) sunflower seeds
1 cup (160 g) raw almonds
¼ cup (35 g) hazelnuts, roughly chopped
¼ cup (40 g) pepitas
¼ cup (60 ml) maple syrup
2½ tablespoons olive oil
1 teaspoon vanilla bean paste or extract
½ teaspoon sea salt

1. Preheat the oven to 350°F (180°C) and line two baking sheets with parchment paper.
2. Mix the sunflower seeds, almonds, hazelnuts, and pepitas together in a bowl, and add the maple syrup, oil, vanilla, and salt. Mix well.
3. Divide the nut mixture between the two baking sheets and spread it evenly over each. Bake for 10 minutes. Then, use a spoon to gently mix the granola on the baking sheets. Swap the baking sheets, from the top to the bottom shelf, to make sure the heat is distributed evenly and the granola is uniformly browned.
4. Continue cooking for another 10 minutes or so, until the granola is crunchy and golden.
5. Serve the granola warm from the oven or at room temperature, but whatever you do, allow the remaining granola to cool completely before transferring it to an airtight container. It keeps well for up to 7 days.

Cacao, Turmeric, and Ginger Smoothie

For a town whose welcome sign reads "Slow down, chill out," Byron Bay, New South Wales, seems to be a few streets ahead of everyone else in a culinary sense. I first tried this flavor combination at a sleepy little café just outside Byron, and I've been replicating it ever since. Ginger, my gastroenterologist tells me, is great for nausea, and also potentially for the underlying causes of said nausea, and turmeric is an anti-inflammatory. Using tahini is a delightful way to add an exotic nutty flavor to smoothies (and basically everything else) without adding any nut butter. It's considered a low-FODMAP food in amounts up to 1 tablespoon, so go nuts (without the nuts, and without exceeding that recommended serving).

1 frozen banana (use an unripe banana if you are particularly sensitive to oligo fructans)

2 teaspoons tahini

2 teaspoons cacao powder

1 teaspoon grated fresh ginger, or to taste

½ to 1 teaspoon fresh turmeric paste or ½ teaspoon ground turmeric

½ cup (125 ml) almond milk, plus a little more, if needed

Optional extras

2½ tablespoons protein powder

A single shot of freshly brewed espresso

2 teaspoons rose water

Ice

1. Place all the ingredients (including your desired optional extras) into a blender and blitz until smooth and creamy.
2. Pour into a glass, and enjoy.

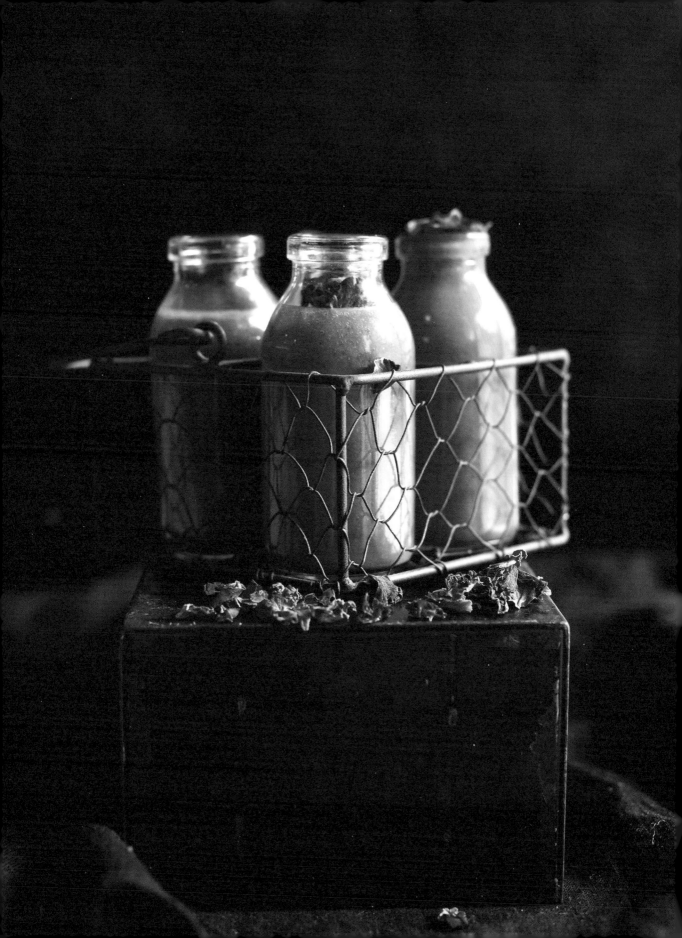

Coconut Rice Bibimbap

When people reference the finer things in life, I'm reasonably certain they're talking about coconut rice. I derive an untold level of happiness from eating a plain bowl of the stuff, but here, I've paired it with bibimbap-inspired toppings, in turn inspired by a pastel-colored brunch spot in New York called Café Henrie.

Coconut rice

1 cup (200 g) jasmine rice
1 cup (250 ml) coconut milk
2 makrut lime leaves (optional)

Quick or slow pickles (fills a 750 ml to 1 L glass jar)

½ cup (125 ml) rice wine vinegar
½ cup (125 ml) apple cider vinegar
¼ cup (25 g) light brown sugar, not packed
1 to 2 teaspoons finely grated fresh ginger
1 to 2 teaspoons sea salt
3 star anise
½ teaspoon cloves
2 bay leaves
2½ cups (300 g) julienned carrots
2½ cups (300 g) thinly sliced cucumbers

Toppings

Fresh carrot, cucumber, and red cabbage (or other low-FODMAP veg of your choice)
4 eggs
Peanut or coconut oil, for frying
1 ripe avocado, thinly sliced
Furikake (see page 119)
Sauerkraut (red cabbage sauerkraut is lower in FODMAPs than the white cabbage version)
Fresh cilantro leaves, chopped (optional)
Fresh red chile, thinly sliced (optional)

1. To make the coconut rice, pour the rice into a large saucepan and add the coconut milk and lime leaves (if using) along with 1½ cups (375 ml) water. Place the saucepan over medium heat and cook for 15 to 20 minutes, until the rice has absorbed the majority of the liquid, stirring intermittently to ensure it isn't sticking to the bottom of the pan. Once the liquid has almost completely absorbed, take the saucepan off the heat and place a lid on it. Allow it to stand for 15 to 20 minutes—it will still be warm, but in this time it will absorb the remaining liquid.

2. Meanwhile, to make the pickles, combine the vinegars, sugar, ginger, salt, spices, and 1 cup (250 ml) water in a medium saucepan. Cook over medium heat until the sugar has dissolved (5 to 10 minutes), and then add the carrot. Cook for 5 to 10 minutes, until the carrot starts to soften. Add the cucumber and cook for a minute or so, until it, too, begins to soften. Remove from the heat.

3. To prepare the toppings, slice your chosen vegetables. Fry the eggs to your liking in a little of the oil.

4. To assemble, place a fried egg in the middle of each of four plates and surround it with the rice, pickles, and the remaining toppings. Serve immediately.

Note: The longer you allow the pickles to pickle, if you will, the more delicious they will be. I transfer mine to a sterilized glass jar, allow them to cool and then put them in the fridge, where they can be kept for months.

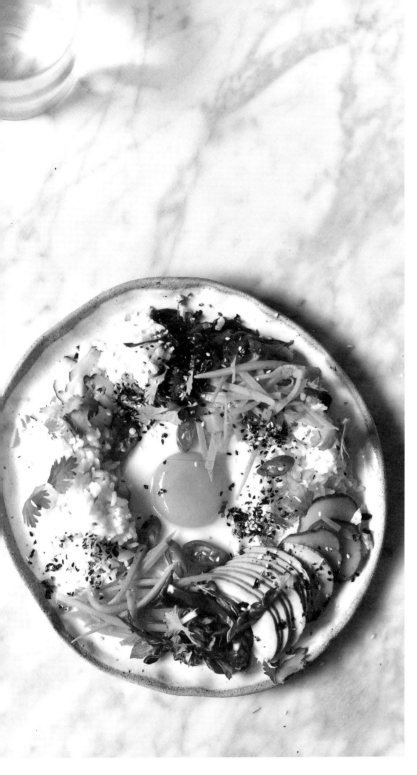

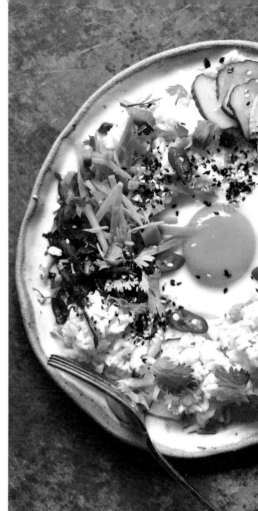

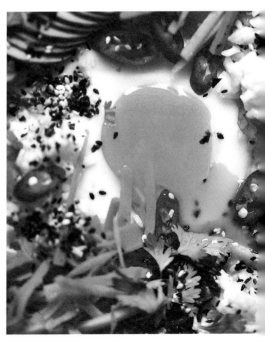

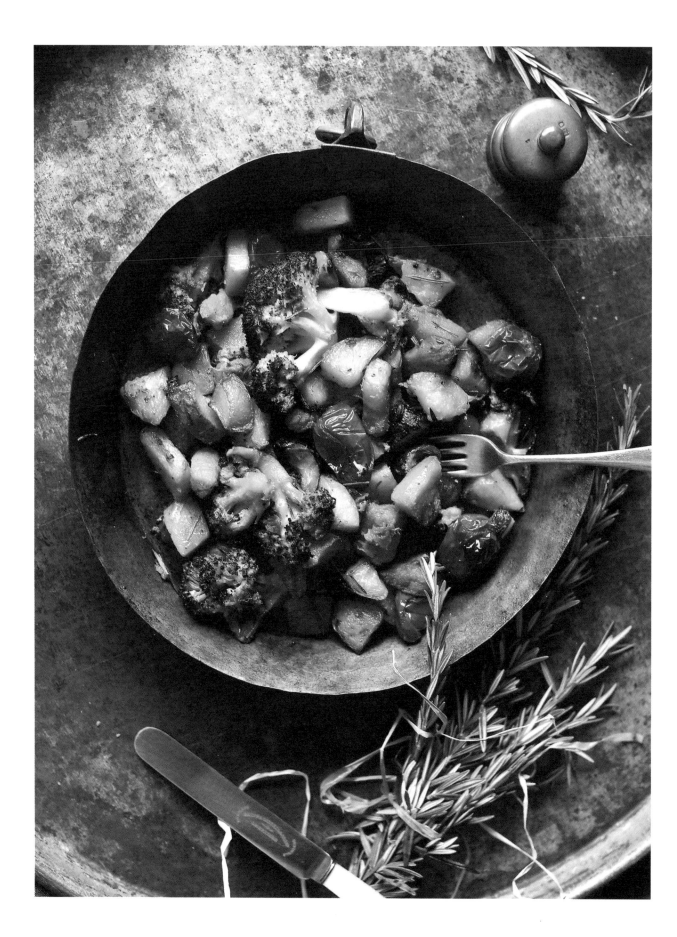

Crispy Sage Breakfast Hash

SERVES 4

As much as I enjoy an extravagant waffle-centric breakfast, sometimes a little simplicity is necessary. I like to keep a batch of this hash in the fridge to have for breakfast (alone or in a scramble, or topped with a fried egg), or tossed through a salad for lunch.

4 cups (1 L) FODMAP-friendly vegetable stock (such as My Go-To Veggie Stock, page 62)

2⅔ cups (400 g) diced small waxy potatoes

1¼ cups (250 g) peeled, diced kabocha squash

5 or 6 sprigs rosemary (optional)

2⅔ cups (200 g) broccoli florets

1 medium (200 g) chopped zucchini

2 tablespoons olive oil or ghee

Small handful of sage leaves, roughly chopped

⅔ cup (100 g) cherry tomatoes

Sea salt and cracked black pepper

1. Pour the stock into a large saucepan and bring to a boil over high heat. Add the potato, squash, and rosemary (if using) and cook for 5 to 10 minutes, until the vegetables are beginning to soften. Add the broccoli and zucchini and continue to cook for another 5 minutes. Once the vegetables are cooked, remove from the heat and strain.

2. Place a large nonstick saucepan over medium heat. Pour in the oil and, once warmed, add the sage leaves and cook for 2 to 3 minutes, until crispy, slightly shriveled, and darkened. They add a beautiful crunch and herbaceous flavor.

3. Add the tomatoes and strained vegetables, along with the rosemary sprigs, if using. Season with salt and pepper.

4. Turn the heat up to high and allow the vegetables to form golden crusts, stirring intermittently. Once they've achieved your desired level of crunchiness, remove from the pan and discard the rosemary sprigs.

Chocolate, Zucchini, and Espresso Muffins

MAKES 12 MUFFINS

Lamenting the stress that is finding time for a vegetable-packed breakfast and a coffee in morning rush hour? No worries, fam. I got you. These muffins are an easy breakfast on the run, combining some of my favorite things: strong espresso, zucchini, and chocolate, at seemingly inappropriate hours of the day.

Muffins

¾ cup (80 g) cocoa powder
2 cups (200 g) almond meal
½ cup (60 g) tapioca flour
1¼ cups (150 g) roughly chopped zucchini
3½ tablespoons (50 g) butter
¼ cup (60 g) almond butter
¼ cup (60 ml) maple syrup
¼ cup (50 g) coconut sugar
2 eggs, lightly beaten
2 tablespoons plus 2 teaspoons coconut oil
½ cup (125 ml) almond milk
2 tablespoons plus 2 teaspoons freshly made espresso
2 teaspoons baking powder
1 tablespoon apple cider vinegar

Icing

2½ tablespoons freshly made espresso
¼ cup (60 ml) melted coconut oil
2½ tablespoons almond butter
2 teaspoons maple syrup
2½ tablespoons cacao powder
Pinch of sea salt (optional)

1. To make the muffins, preheat the oven to 350°F (180°C). Lightly grease a 12-cup muffin pan (you can use muffin liners, too, if you like).

2. Combine all the muffin ingredients in a food processor (add the cocoa first so it doesn't fly everywhere when you start mixing) and process into a smooth, dark chocolaty mixture. Divide evenly between the muffin cups. Bake for 20 minutes, or until a skewer inserted into the center of a muffin comes out clean.

3. Allow the muffins to cool for a couple of minutes before running a knife around the edge of each cup. Transfer the muffins to a wire rack and allow them to cool completely before icing—a difficult but necessary step, as coconut oil–based icing is notorious for melting.

4. Meanwhile, to make the icing, mix the espresso, oil, almond butter, and maple syrup together, until it has formed a mostly smooth liquid (don't be alarmed by the few grainy bits from the almond butter). Stir in the cacao until all the lumps are gone. Spread on the cooled muffins and add a pinch of salt, if you like.

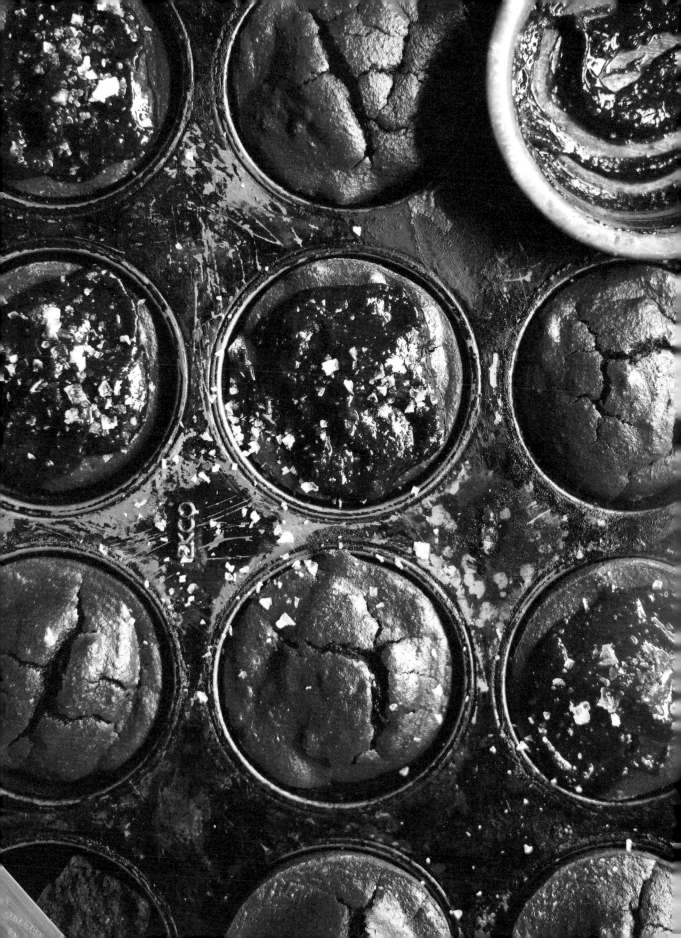

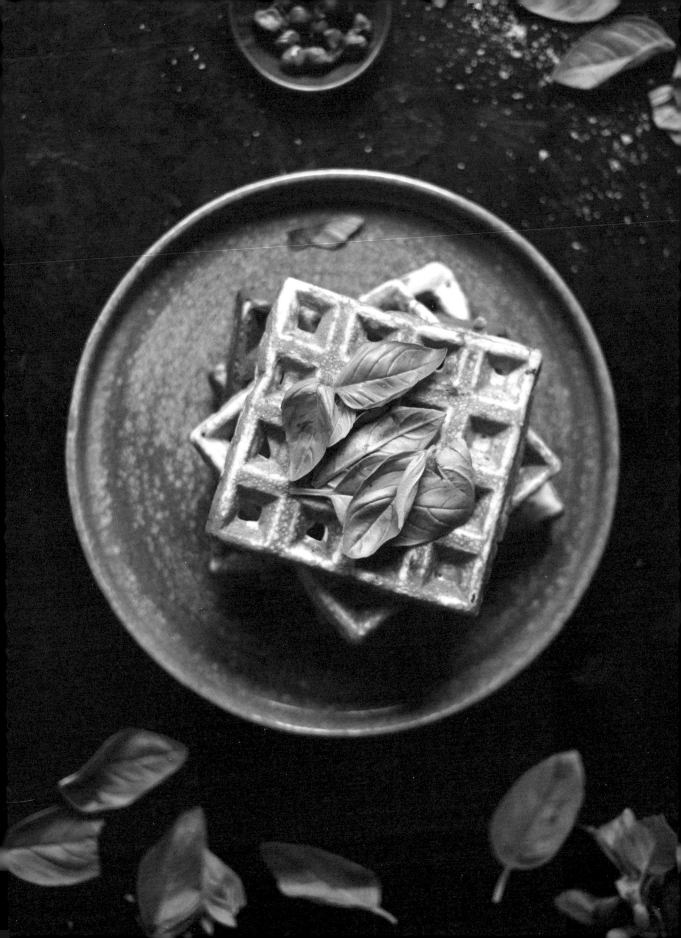

Buckwheat, Parmesan, and Caper Waffles

SERVES 2

Although the majority of Instagram glory seems to be found in over-sweetened and overdecorated breakfast foods, I have always been, and always will be, a savory girl first. I personally find that sweet breakfasts set me up for a day of craving sugar, which, when you spend your life recipe testing and often surrounded by cake, is not ideal. These savory numbers are dead easy to make, and have all the glory of a waffle, without leaving me feeling like I *need* to eat half a cake later in the day. Serve them as they are, or with a poached egg and some soft herbs scattered on top (I like basil or dill).

¾ cup (90 g) buckwheat flour
¼ cup (30 g) tapioca flour
1½ teaspoons baking powder
2 eggs
1 tablespoon olive oil
¾ cup (180 ml) lactose-free milk
½ cup (50 g) finely grated
   vegetarian Parmesan
3 tablespoons caper berries or
   capers, chopped
2 teaspoons apple cider vinegar
Neutral oil spray

1. Mix all of the ingredients together in a bowl until well combined.
2. Preheat a waffle maker.
3. Spray the heated waffle maker lightly with oil and pour a quarter of the mixture into each iron. Cook for 3 to 5 minutes, until the waffles are golden brown and smell delicious. Serve warm.

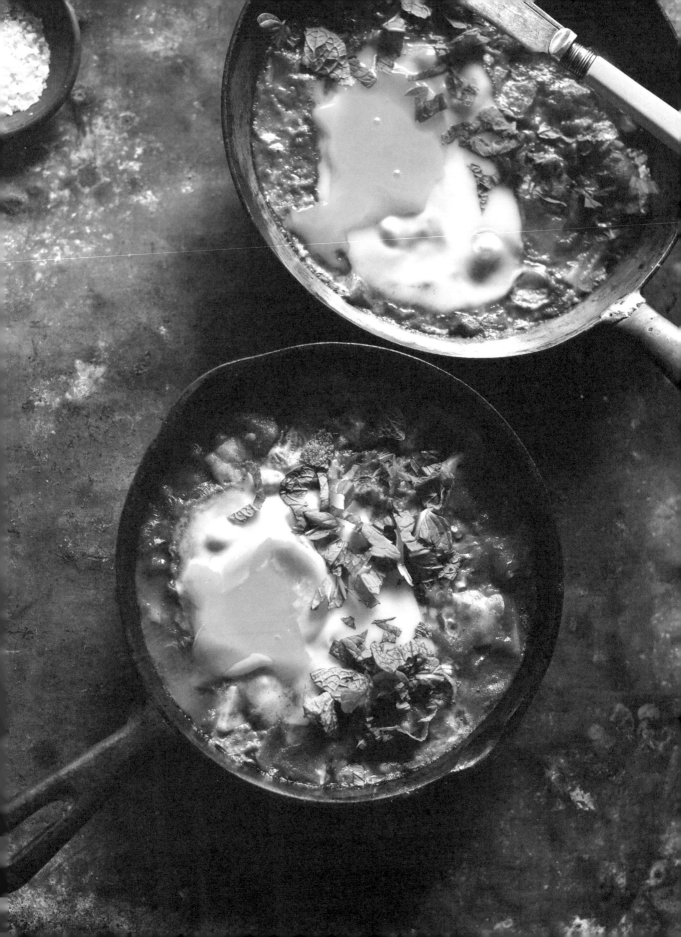

Roasted Pepper and Halloumi Shakshuka

Since the volume of onion and garlic in a standard restaurant shakshuka could put me in bed for a week, I've given up ordering baked eggs when I'm out in favor of making them at home. Although they're a little labor intensive, roasted peppers are a great substitute for the sweetness of caramelized onion, and anything that includes halloumi warrants a bit of extra elbow grease, as far as I'm concerned.

4 medium-large red bell peppers
2½ tablespoons olive oil
2 pounds (1 kg) tomatoes, chopped
2 teaspoons ground cumin
1 teaspoon pumpkin pie spice
1 teaspoon garam masala
2 teaspoons light brown sugar
1 teaspoon harissa or hot sauce (make sure it doesn't contain onion or garlic)
1 teaspoon tomato paste
½ piece (10 to 15 g) preserved lemon rind
4 ounces (125 g) halloumi, diced
Handful each of fresh mint and cilantro leaves, or your preferred herb, plus extra to garnish
Juice of ½ lemon
4 eggs

1. Preheat the oven to 350°F (180°C) and line a baking sheet with parchment paper.
2. Slice the peppers in half, remove the seeds, and lay them face down on the baking sheet. Cook for at least 30 minutes, or until the flesh is soft and the skin has blistered and blackened. Transfer them to a large bowl and cover with a cloth, to encourage them to sweat their skins off (aka what happens to me whenever the temperature reaches 80°F/26°C or higher). Peel off the skins and roughly chop.
3. Heat the oil and tomatoes in a cast-iron frying pan over medium heat (or you can use four small pans if you have them). Adding water as you see fit, cook the tomatoes down until they have the consistency of pasta sauce. Add the spices, sugar, harissa, tomato paste, and preserved lemon and gently stir to combine. Add the peppers, halloumi, herbs, and lemon juice and stir gently to disperse throughout the mixture.
4. Using the back of a spoon, create a little indent for each egg, and gently crack one into each well. Turn the heat down to low and cook extremely gently for a few minutes, alternating between placing a lid on and taking it off. Once the whites are cooked but the yolks still slightly runny, remove the pan from the heat and top with more herbs and additional seasoning, as desired.
5. Allow to sit for a couple of minutes, so your guests don't burn their hands on the pan or their mouths on the shakshuka.

Carrot, Parsnip, and Parmesan Latkes

MAKES AROUND
6 LATKES
(enough for 2 to
3 people)

A statement that will either make me sound like a plebe or encourage us to become best friends: These latkes taste a lot like cheesy hash browns, which is entirely why I'm so fond of them. Although the traditional variety is made with potato, I've used carrot and parsnip, two lesser-worshipped, but equally delicious, FODMAP-friendly vegetables. These latkes are free of gluten, grains, and nuts, low in lactose, and suitable for almost all dietary requirements under the sun. Serve the latkes on their own, or topped with a fried egg and herbs scattered on top.

1 cup (100 g) grated parsnips
1 cup (100 g) grated carrots
1 teaspoon salt
¾ cup (75 g) freshly grated
    vegetarian Parmesan
1 egg
Cracked black pepper
1 tablespoon roughly chopped
    soft herbs (dill or mint work
    well)
Neutral oil with a high smoke
    point (I use vegetable oil)

1. Scoop the grated vegetables into a cheesecloth, nut milk bag, or clean, non-white tea towel. Sprinkle with the salt and allow to sit over the sink in a colander for 10 minutes. Using considerable force, wring the water out of the vegetables, and then transfer to a medium bowl.

2. Add the Parmesan and egg and mix thoroughly until a rough batter has formed. Add a good sprinkle of pepper, and the herbs, if you are using them.

3. Heat a nonstick frying pan over medium-high heat and add enough of the oil to completely cover the bottom of the pan. Allow the oil to heat up thoroughly before adding a tablespoon or two of the latke mixture. Use the back of a spoon to press it down firmly and create a thin latke, about the size of your palm. Cook for a few minutes before gently flipping. The latke should be golden brown and crunchy on the outside.

4. Repeat with the remaining mixture and serve warm.

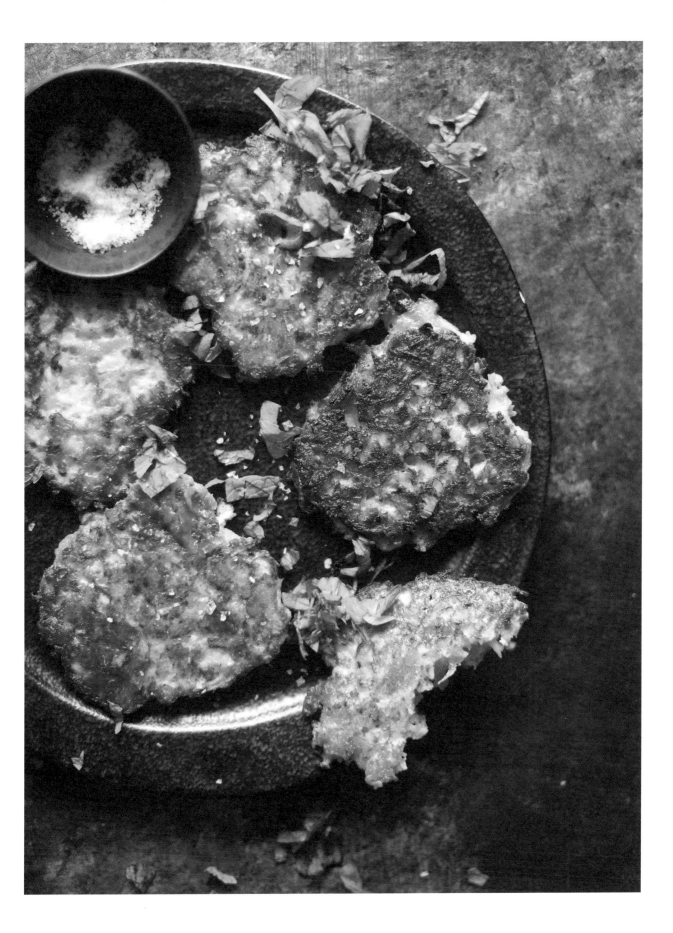

Savory Brown Rice Crepes with Curried Potato

SERVES 4

These savory crepes taste a bit like dosa (although they're not fermented or nearly as artful), so they pair like a dream with curried potato. Through the years, I've learned that the singular perk of being unable to eat onion and garlic is that there's zero possibility of winding up with garlic breath first thing in the morning. In other words, you're free to eat curried potato breakfasts with reckless abandon. Hey, silver lining, I see you.

Curried potato

1½ pounds (750 g) small waxy potatoes, peeled and diced into small, even pieces (about 5 cups)

2 tablespoons ghee or butter

2 teaspoons ground turmeric

1 teaspoon coriander seeds

1 teaspoon garam masala

½ teaspoon sea salt

½ teaspoon ground cumin

1½ teaspoons finely grated fresh ginger

Fresh red chile or red pepper flakes, to taste (make sure to seed and finely chop if you're using fresh), plus extra for garnish

Savory crepes

½ cup (65 g) fine brown rice flour

2 teaspoons tapioca flour

1 egg

¾ cup (180 ml) milk of your choice

½ teaspoon fine salt

Butter or ghee, for frying (I find butter does a better job for crepes)

To serve

Greek or coconut yogurt

Small handful of fresh cilantro leaves

1. **To make the curried potato,** steam the potatoes gently over boiling water for about 10 minutes, until they are soft and cooked through. Remove from the heat and leave to steam dry for a few minutes.

2. Gently heat the ghee in a large frying pan over medium-low heat. Add the turmeric, coriander, garam masala, salt, and cumin and cook for a few minutes until they become fragrant. Add the ginger and chile and cook for an additional minute or so.

3. Add the potato and turn the heat to high. Fry until the potatoes are golden, smoking, and covered in the spices, about 5 to 10 minutes.

4. **Meanwhile, to make the crepes,** whisk all the ingredients in a large bowl until a batter forms.

5. Heat a crepe pan or medium nonstick frying pan over medium-high heat and melt a little butter. Tilt and swirl the pan to evenly coat the bottom.

6. Pour about ¼ cup (60 ml) of the batter into the pan and use your wrist to swirl the batter around until you get your desired shape (or undesired shape—practice makes perfect, right?). Allow to cook and bubble for a minute or so, keeping an eye on it. When the mixture looks solid on top, flip it over and cook on the other side for another minute.

7. Transfer to a plate, cover to keep warm, and repeat the process until you're out of batter.

8. **To serve,** divide the hot curried potato evenly between the crepes and then top with a spoonful of yogurt and some cilantro and chile.

Sweet Quinoa and Lemon Crepes

MAKES 6 TO
8 CREPES

I was at university by the time I "discovered" crepes, and by that point, I'd already stopped eating gluten, so I didn't really discover them at all. My school had a "campus famous" crepe stand, and one night I met a cute medical student who asked me out for crepes. Too awkward to tell him I was unable to eat crepes, I avoided him for the rest of my degree. Am I overcompensating for the depth of my awkward personality by including two different gluten-free recipes for crepes in this book? I'll let you decide.

½ cup (65 g) quinoa flour
¾ cup (180 ml) milk of your choice
1 tablespoon maple syrup
1 teaspoon vanilla bean paste or extract
Zest of 1 lemon
1 egg
Butter, for frying

To serve
Maple syrup
A few lemon wedges

1. Whisk together the flour, milk, maple syrup, vanilla, lemon zest, and egg in a medium bowl until combined.
2. Heat a crepe pan or medium nonstick frying pan over medium-high heat and melt a small amount of butter. Using your wrist to tilt the pan, swirl the butter around the pan to evenly coat the bottom.
3. Pour about ¼ cup (60 ml) of the batter into the pan and, using that fancy wrist technique, swirl it around until you get your desired shape.
4. Cook until the top of the crepe is just starting to solidify, then flip over and cook for another 30 seconds to a minute on the other side.
5. Transfer the crepe to a plate and then repeat the process by greasing the pan and adding more batter. Continue until you have used up all the mixture.
6. Serve with a drizzle of maple syrup and a good squeeze of lemon juice.

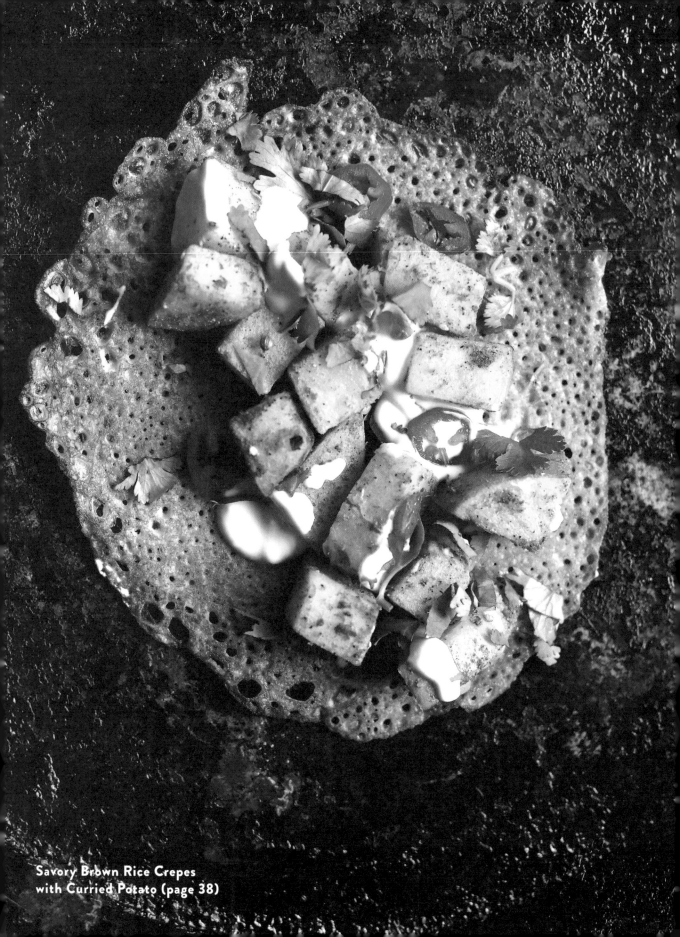

Savory Brown Rice Crepes
with Curried Potato (page 38)

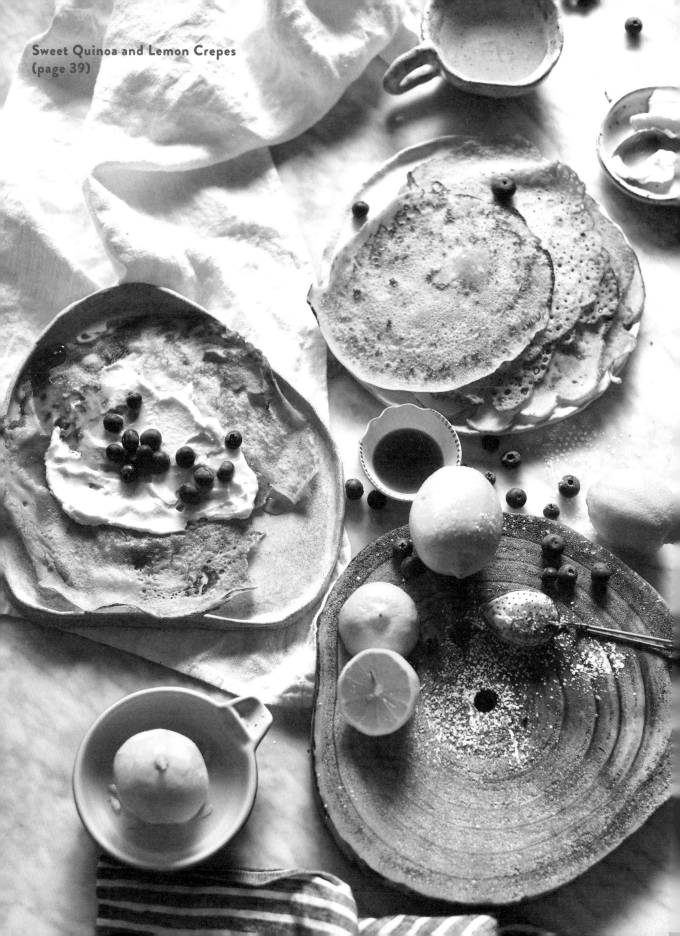

Sweet Quinoa and Lemon Crepes
(page 39)

Roasted Quinoa and Banana Crumble

Before you @ me re: bananas, let's have a tolerant discussion about intolerance. Firstly, not every FODMAPper has an issue with fructans, the main issue with bananas. Secondly, an underripe banana is (at the time of writing) considered FODMAP friendly in servings of one banana at a time. Thirdly, you're not tied to bananas! Use rhubarb or strawberries for a lower-FODMAP but equally delicious option. Serve this with coconut yogurt and Nutella or melted dark chocolate. Or, you know, whatever the hell you want to serve it with.

4 small or 2 large underripe bananas (or other fruit of choice)

¼ cup (25 g) quinoa flakes

2½ tablespoons tapioca flour

1 tablespoon light brown sugar

½ teaspoon baking powder

½ teaspoon vanilla bean paste or extract

2 tablespoons (30 g) good-quality butter, room temperature

½ teaspoon spice of your choice (optional; I'm looking at you, cinnamon or nutmeg)

1. Preheat the oven to 350°F (180°C).
2. Gently peel and slice the bananas lengthwise (I hold the curve of the bare banana in my hand and gently slice from the top down, longest side of the banana first) and place them on a baking sheet lined with parchment paper. Bake for 20 minutes or until golden and cooked through but still firm-ish.
3. Mix the quinoa flakes, tapioca flour, sugar, and baking powder together in a small bowl, add the vanilla, and use your hands to rub the butter into the mixture, until it is crumbly but still in solid form (rather than melty butter).
4. Arrange the cooked bananas in a small ovenproof vessel of your choosing and sprinkle the crumble over the top. Keep in mind that the crumble spreads, in the event that you want to see banana in the finished product. I get it. Aesthetics.
5. Place the crumble in the oven for 10 to 15 minutes, depending on how crisp you like your crumble. Serve warm.

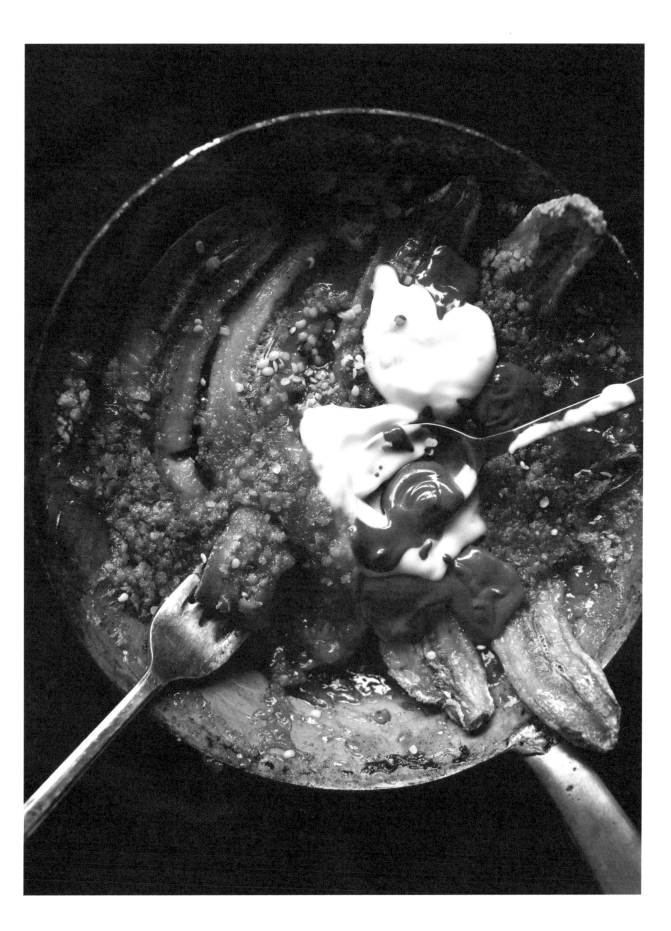

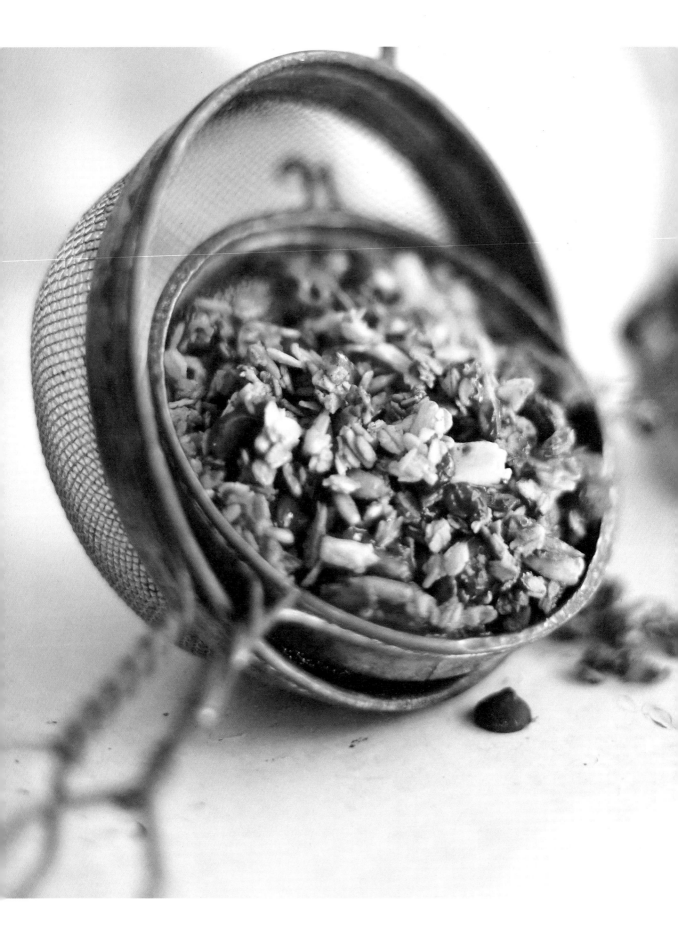

Oat and Chocolate Chip Granola

MAKES 5 CUPS
(550 G)

I know I mentioned earlier in this chapter that I like to keep granola simple, but I'm reasonably certain that contradiction is the spice of life, not variety. Whatever the case, this granola is overwhelmingly simple to make but tastes just a little bit extravagant. You can serve the granola with milk, on coconut yogurt, on smoothie bowls . . . or, you know, just eat it out of the jar. Hot tip: You can make this vegan by substituting the butter and chocolate with dairy-free alternatives, and nut-free by replacing the cup of nuts with more seeds and some coconut flakes.

7 tablespoons (100 g) butter

¼ cup (60 ml) maple syrup

1 tablespoon coconut sugar or light brown sugar

1 teaspoon vanilla bean paste or extract

½ teaspoon salt

Cinnamon or nutmeg (optional)

1 cup (140 g) nuts of choice (I use half almonds and half peanuts)

1 cup (150 g) sunflower seeds

2 cups (200 g) gluten-free rolled oats (regular oats are also FODMAP-friendly, if you don't need them to be gluten-free)

⅓ cup (50 g) dark chocolate chips

1. Preheat the oven to 350°F (180°C). Line two baking sheets with parchment paper.
2. Melt the butter and mix it with the maple syrup, sugar, vanilla, and salt. You can also add a few pinches of ground cinnamon or nutmeg, if you're in the mood.
3. Mix the nuts, seeds, and oats together in a large bowl. Pour the butter mixture over the top, stirring well to combine.
4. Divide the mixture between the two lined baking sheets and place in the oven for 10 minutes.
5. Swap the trays from top to bottom, rotate them, and use a large spoon to gently mix the granola. Bake for another 10 minutes.
6. Allow the granola to cool for about 15 minutes before tossing in the chocolate chips. They will melt slightly and form delicious chunks of chocolate and granola.

Lactose-Free "Ricotta" Toasts

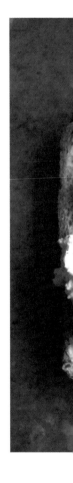

MAKES
APPROXIMATELY 1 CUP
(250 G) "RICOTTA";
each toast recipe serves 1

Ricotta on toast is a delightfully blank slate to which you can apply almost anything—honey and peanut butter, radicchio and balsamic, peas and mint. Almost as delightful is the fact that you can use this recipe anywhere you'd use regular ricotta (the Involtini on page 106, for example)—just be aware you might get through a bit of lactose-free milk in the process.

Ricotta
4 cups (1 L) lactose-free whole milk
¼ cup (60 ml) lemon juice (you can also use white vinegar or apple cider vinegar, but they will leave more of an aftertaste)
1 teaspoon fine salt, or to taste

Balsamic Radicchio Toasts
2 slices gluten-free bread
FODMAP-Friendly Pesto (page 121)
Radicchio, chopped
Sea salt flakes and freshly cracked pepper, to taste
Drizzle of balsamic vinegar, to taste

Pea and Mint Toasts
2 slices gluten-free bread
FODMAP-Friendly Pesto (page 121)
1 to 2 tablespoons peas
Mint, chopped
1 to 2 tablespoons toasted pine nuts
Red pepper flakes (optional)

1. To make the ricotta, combine the milk and salt in a large saucepan over medium-low heat. Allow the milk to come to a simmer, 10 to 15 minutes. Turn the heat off and move the pan well away from any heat.

2. Add the lemon juice. Stir gently, only to distribute the acid in the milk. Allow to sit for 15 minutes—the mixture should have curdled and become obvious "curds and whey." There should be ricotta-like lumps of milk and a semi-transparent lemon-colored liquid. If the liquid is still milky and completely opaque, return the ricotta to a gentle heat until it begins to separate, and then take it off the heat again to rest for 15 minutes. You can add a little extra lemon juice (a teaspoon at a time) as an insurance policy, although this might affect the taste of the final product.

3. Gently pour the ricotta through a sieve lined with cheesecloth or a nut milk bag. You can discard the whey or use it in smoothies or baking (see Notes for a few more ideas). How long you strain the ricotta is up to you—it depends on how runny you like it. I like mine on the more spreadable side, so I either give it a good old squeeze and decant, or strain it for a maximum of 20 minutes. If you prefer a drier ricotta, leave it to drain for 30 minutes or longer. If you accidentally overstrain, you can add a little lactose-free milk to loosen it up.

4. To make this more spreadable, simply whip the ricotta in a stand mixer or with a hand mixer, until it is light and fluffy. Season to taste with more salt or add in any flavorings you see fit.

5. To make the toasts, spread the whipped ricotta over freshly toasted gluten-free bread and top with the accompaniments of your choice. Store any leftover ricotta in an airtight container. This keeps for a few days in the fridge.

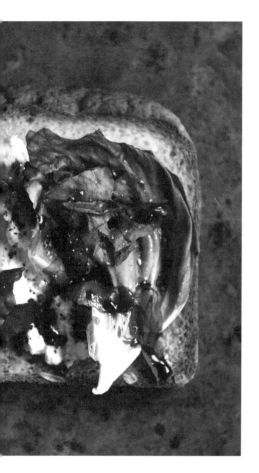

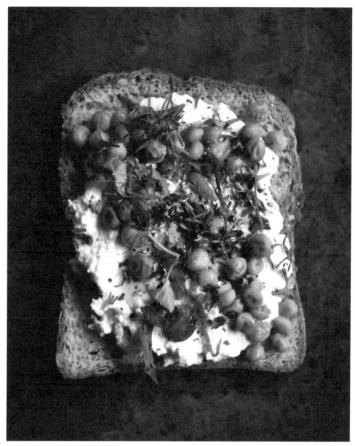

Note: Ricotta is quite a high-lactose and FODMAP cheese, so this version is a great alternative for those with a lactose intolerance or on a FODMAP diet. This ricotta is delicious plain but can also be flavored with whatever you fancy—herbs, a bit of balsamic, truffle oil, or a smoked salt. You can use the leftover acidic liquid in smoothies, pizza crusts, curries—basically any cooking process that requires liquid. It adds a unique tang and a bunch of nutrients from the milk. And, of course, full-fat lactose-free milk creates a better lactose-free ricotta. Period.

Green Bread

I'd tell you that I'm not a huge bread eater, but **80 percent of what's on the gluten-free market barely passes as bread. With that (bitterly) in mind, I went ahead and made my own bright green, herbaceous version. This bread pairs well with most savory accompaniments, but my favorite is some FODMAP-Friendly Pesto (page 121), sliced tomato, and sea salt. This mixture also makes excellent green pancakes.**

1 cup (100 g) grated zucchini (skin on)

1½ teaspoons fine salt

2 large bunches basil (100 g), washed and roughly chopped

4 ounces (100 g) baby spinach leaves, washed and roughly chopped

¼ cup (60 ml) boiling water

½ cup (50 g) freshly and finely grated vegetarian Parmesan

2 eggs

1¼ cup (125 g) almond meal

¾ cup (100 g) fine white rice flour

½ cup (60 g) tapioca flour

¼ cup (60 ml) almond milk

2 teaspoons baking powder

1 tablespoon apple cider vinegar

1. Preheat the oven to 350°F (180°C). Place a silicone loaf pan on a baking sheet and lightly grease the pan.

2. Place the zucchini in a fine mesh sieve with 1 teaspoon of the salt. Use your hands to mix together and then set aside. The salt will draw out a significant amount of moisture from the zucchini, so the bread won't be too soggy. Squeeze the zucchini vigorously to remove extra moisture—you should get around ⅓ cup (80 ml). Place the zucchini in a food processor and discard the liquid.

3. Place the basil and spinach in a large bowl. Pour the boiling water over the greens to blanch them. Leave for 15 to 20 seconds before removing. (Any longer and they risk turning brown.) Once they have drained and cooled, use your hands to vigorously wring them out as you did the zucchini, to prevent the loaf from becoming soggy. Transfer to the food processor.

4. Add the Parmesan and blend until a smooth, vibrant green paste has formed. Providing the mixture isn't too hot, add the eggs, almond meal, flours, milk, and the remaining ½ teaspoon salt, and blend to combine.

5. Pour the mixture into a large bowl and add the baking powder and vinegar. Stir to combine. The mixture should appear bubbly and almost fluffy. Pour it into the greased loaf pan atop the baking sheet and then bake in the oven for 40 to 45 minutes. Note that wet spots can be present in the middle of the loaf even when ostensibly cooked, so leave it in the oven for extra time if in doubt. You'll know it's done when a skewer comes out clean.

6. Allow to cool slightly before gently removing it from the loaf pan and placing onto a cooling rack. Cool before slicing. Keep the loaf in an airtight contained for around 4 days, or slice and freeze.

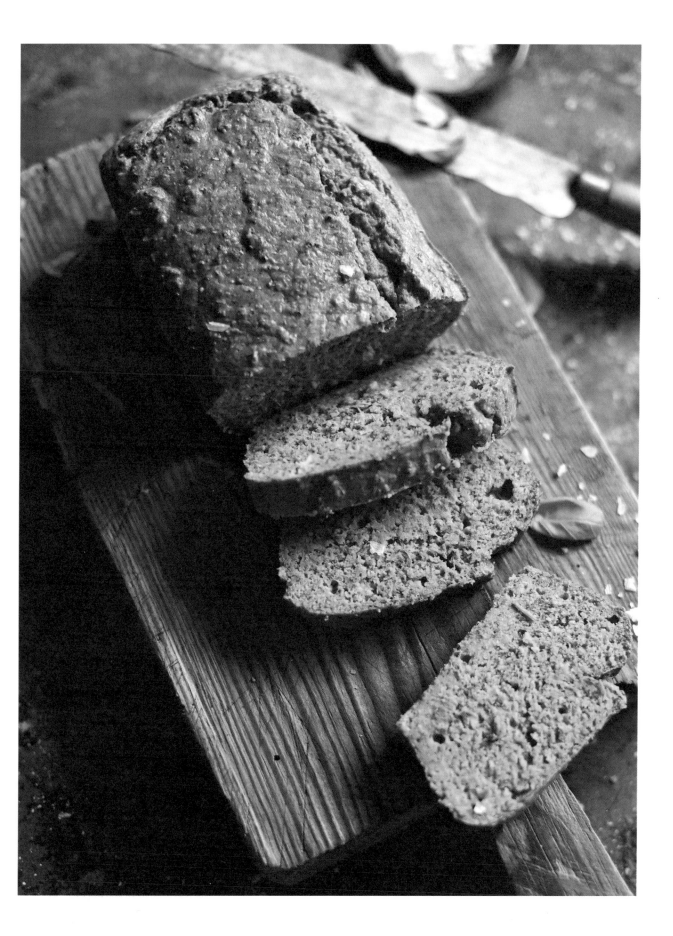

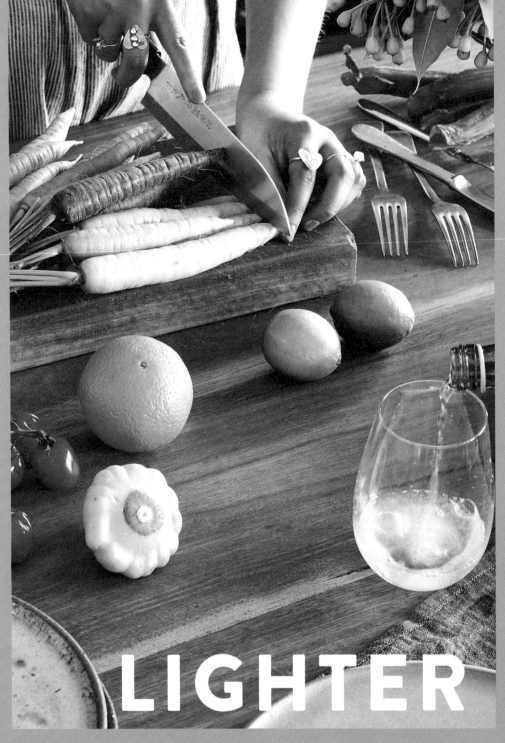

LIGHTER RECIPES

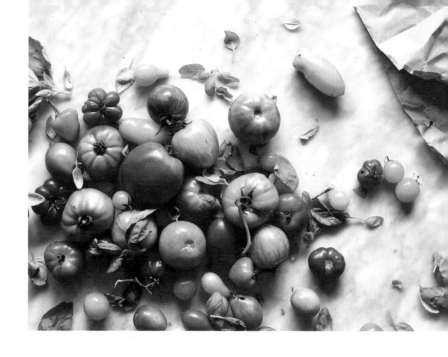

Although I'm unconvinced that I've ever eaten what could be considered "a lighter meal," I can concede that sometimes less is more. That's why I have created a chapter of lighter meals—for those moments when dinner is too much but a handful of olives while staring listlessly at the fridge is too little.

This chapter contains everything from salt and vinegar potatoes to vegetarian or vegan Caesar salads, from blood orange salads to bread ones.

These are meals appropriate for a work lunch, a dinner party side, a light lunch or heavy snack, and everything in between.

Sweet and Sticky Buckwheat Noodles with Quick Crispy Tofu

That the word *sticky* suddenly becomes desirous when talking about something with *sweet* or *noodle* in the title never ceases to amaze me. Other things that amaze me? The ease and deliciousness of this recipe (you saw that one coming, surely). It's gluten-free, vegan, ready in twenty, and endlessly customizable. Use whichever vegetables are in season/you have on hand/you prefer. Use rice noodles if you can't find 100 percent buckwheat ones—(almost) anything goes.

Sweet and sticky sauce

½ cup (120 ml) white rice vinegar
¼ cup (60 ml) gluten-free tamari
¼ cup (60 ml) pure maple syrup (check that it's 100 percent maple)
Generous grating of fresh ginger (1 to 2 packed teaspoons)

Crispy tofu

10 ounces (300 g) firm tofu, pressed (see Note on page 119) and cubed
1 tablespoon gluten-free cornstarch
Sesame seeds and sea salt (optional)

To finish

8 ounces (250 g) 100 percent buckwheat noodles
Toasted sesame oil
2½ tablespoons refined sesame oil
1 bunch radishes (including tops)
1 bunch small carrots (including tops)
1 bunch bok choy
Black or white sesame seeds, lightly toasted
Fresh chile or red pepper flakes (optional)

1. To make the sauce, combine all the ingredients in a small saucepan over medium-low heat. Cook for about 10 minutes, or until the liquids have thickened slightly and become saucy. Set aside.

2. To make the tofu, place the tofu pieces in a medium bowl and toss them in the cornstarch. Add some sesame seeds and sea salt, if you like.

3. To finish, prepare the noodles according to the instructions on the package. The brand I use is cooked in boiling water. (Some noodles tend to become mush when you do that, however, so read the instructions.) Drain, drizzle liberally with toasted sesame oil (to prevent them from sticking), and cover with a lid, to trap the steam and keep them from drying up.

4. In a large heavy-bottomed saucepan or wok, heat the refined sesame oil over medium-high heat. Add the tofu in batches and cook until each side of the cube is golden. Don't overcrowd the pan or the tofu will become soggy. Place the cooked tofu on a plate to the side.

5. Keeping the wok on medium-high heat, pour in the sauce. It will bubble and spit, so be careful. Allow it to thicken for a minute or so.

6. Depending on how cooked you like your veg, you might want to add the radishes and carrots now; otherwise, add them with the other vegetables. Add the noodles, gently breaking them up with a fork.

7. Add the radishes and carrots with their greens, the bok choy, and the tofu and gently toss to coat. Once cooked to your liking (be aware that buckwheat noodles can be fickle, so don't overcook them), remove from the heat.

8. Sprinkle with toasted sesame seeds and chile, if using, drizzle with more toasted sesame oil, and serve.

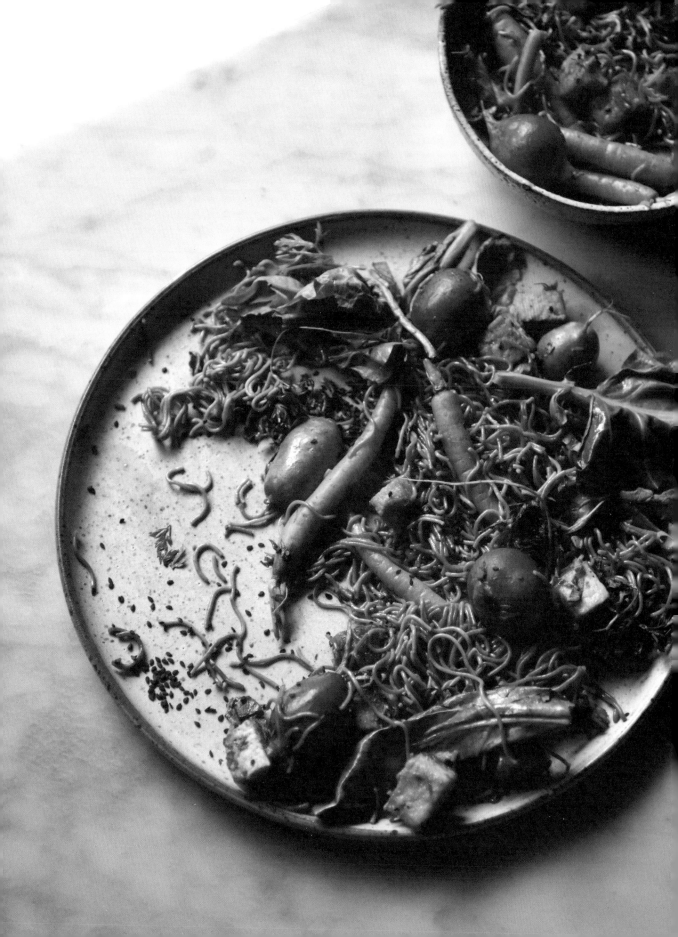

Roasted Dukkah Carrots with Fennel Salad

SERVES 4
as a side

Much like me and the musician Flume, carrots, dukkah, and goat cheese are meant to be together. I've paired them with fennel instead of the usual salad greens to bring a bit of freshness and crunch to an otherwise richly flavored dish. In servings under a cup, fennel is a great low-FODMAP vegetable to get on board with, which puts it in the same boat as goat cheese, which has a low lactose content.

Roasted carrots

1 pound (500 g) carrots
2½ tablespoons olive oil
1 teaspoon ground cinnamon
1 teaspoon ground cumin
3 to 4 tablespoons Dukkah (page 55), plus extra to serve

Fennel salad

1 fennel bulb; reserve fronds, if there are any
Pinch of sea salt
1 tablespoon extra virgin olive oil
Juice of 1 lemon

To serve

2 to 4 ounces (50 to 100 g) goat cheese
1 small bunch mint leaves, roughly chopped
Lemon wedges

1. Preheat the oven to 350°F (180°C). Line a baking sheet with parchment paper.
2. To make the roasted carrots, chop the carrots into evenly sized batons and pop them on the lined baking sheet. Drizzle with the olive oil. Add the cinnamon, cumin, and dukkah, then toss together really well to coat the carrots.
3. Bake in the oven for 20 to 30 minutes, until the carrots are tender and nicely browned.
4. Meanwhile, to make the fennel salad, cut the ends off the fennel bulb and remove the thick outer layer. Thinly slice the bulb as evenly as you can. (By far the easiest and most efficient way to do this is with a mandoline. If you have one, make sure you use the guard!) Place the slices in a bowl with the salt, extra virgin olive oil, and lemon juice, then toss together.
5. To serve, create a bed of the fennel on a serving plate and arrange the hot roasted carrots on top. Drizzle with any lemony oils left in the fennel bowl. Finish with small pieces of goat cheese crumbled on top, some mint, any reserved fennel fronds, a sprinkle of the dukkah, and some lemon wedges.

Dukkah

MAKES
2 ½ CUPS
(330 G)

Here's a cheap and easy way to get to Melbourne, if you can't afford the airfare: Sprinkle this dukkah on everything you possibly can and serve with an obscure, single-origin coffee. Dukkah is a flavor enhancer when your diet is limited, and it is embarrassingly easy to make. If you don't like macadamias or hazelnuts, you can substitute them for another FODMAP-friendly nut. Cheap and easy, as I said.

¾ cup (100 g) macadamia nuts
¾ cup (100 g) hazelnuts
1 cup (125 g) sesame seeds
2½ teaspoons cumin seeds
2½ teaspoons coriander seeds
½ teaspoon sea salt
½ teaspoon garam masala
½ teaspoon ground turmeric
Pinch of red pepper flakes
    (optional)

1. Preheat the oven to 350°F (180°C). Line a baking sheet with parchment paper.
2. Spread the macadamias and hazelnuts evenly on the lined baking sheet, then place in the oven for 5 to 10 minutes, until the nuts are lovely and brown.
3. Lightly toast the sesame seeds in a frying pan over a medium heat, watching them constantly. They burn easily (much like me in the sun!).
4. Transfer the toasted nuts and sesame seeds to a food processor, along with the remaining ingredients. Pulse until you achieve your desired consistency—I like mine with a few small nut chunks.
5. Store in an airtight jar and use on everything and anything you see fit—scrambled eggs, salads, and roasted vegetables are good places to start. Dukkah keeps well in an airtight container, out of the sunlight, for up to 2 months.

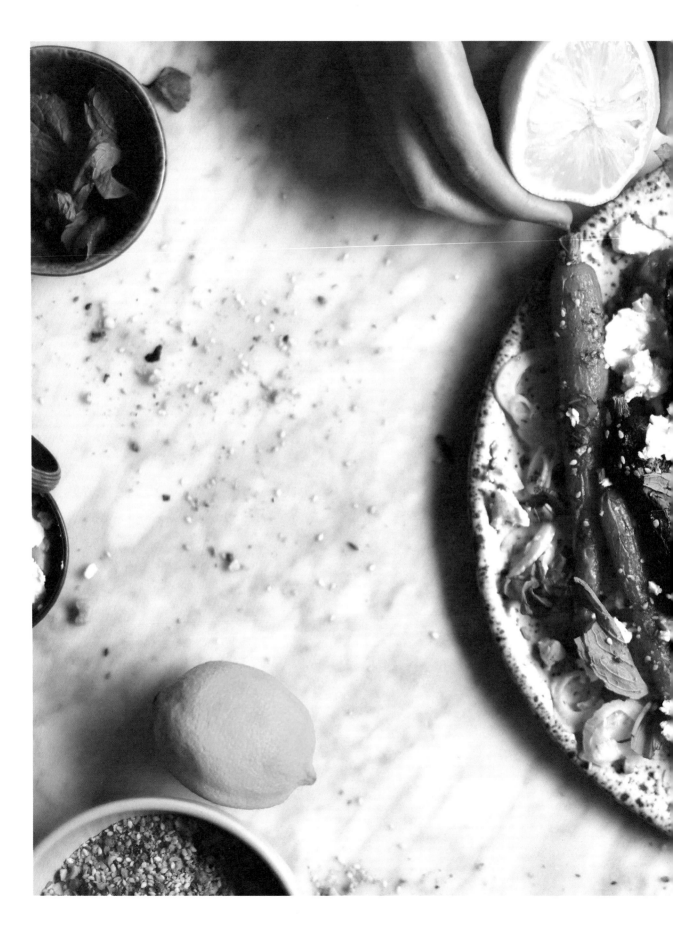

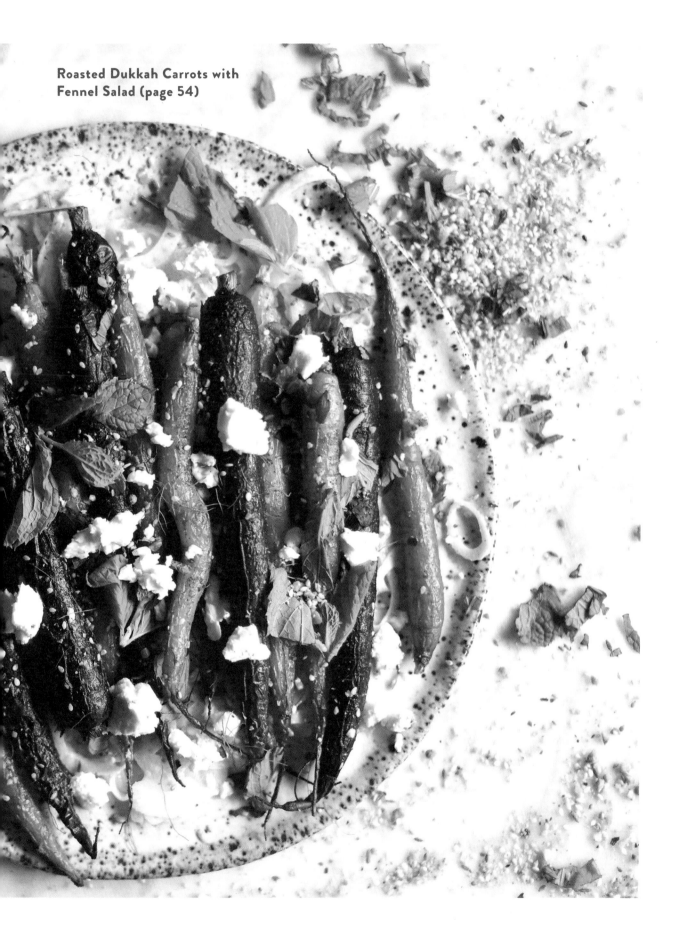

Roasted Dukkah Carrots with
Fennel Salad (page 54)

Quinoa, Fresh Tomato, and Fried Bread Salad

If the words *fried bread salad* don't entice you, then I'm not really sure what will. This salad is the untraditional, FODMAP-friendly love child of tabbouleh and fattoush, two Middle Eastern salads I've had to give up since going low-FODMAP. You can omit the feta or substitute a vegan version if need be, but I cannot condone the omission of the fried bread—it's the highlight of each mouthful.

Quinoa

1 cup (200 g) quinoa

2½ cups (625 ml) FODMAP-friendly vegetable stock (such as My Go-To Veggie Stock, page 62)

½ piece (10 to 15 g) preserved lemon rind

Pinch of sea salt

Fried bread

5 ounces (150 g) gluten-free bread

2 teaspoons olive oil

½ to 1 teaspoon sea salt

½ teaspoon sumac

Fattoush salad

½ bunch mint, roughly chopped, plus extra to garnish

½ bunch flat-leaf parsley or cilantro, roughly chopped, plus extra to garnish

1 pound (450 g) heirloom cherry or grape tomatoes, halved if large

1 red chile, seeded and finely chopped

Sea salt

⅓ to ⅔ cup (50 to 100 g) crumbled feta cheese, depending on your taste and tolerance

Lemon juice

Olive oil

Sumac

1. **To make the quinoa,** combine the quinoa, stock, preserved lemon, and salt in a medium saucepan and bring to a boil over high heat. Lower the heat to medium and continue to cook, stirring intermittently, until the majority of the liquid has evaporated. Once it's nearly all gone and the quinoa tails have unfurled, remove from the heat and cover with a lid for 10 to 15 minutes. This will finish the cooking process without creating mushy quinoa.

2. **To make the fried bread,** chop the bread into small squares and heat a frying pan over medium-high heat. Add the oil, salt, and sumac, and then the bread. Cook, tossing regularly, until the bread is crunchy and brown. Set aside.

3. **To make the fattoush salad,** combine the mint, parsley, tomatoes, chile, and pinch of salt in a large bowl.

4. Add the quinoa and fried bread to the bowl. Garnish with the extra mint and parsley, then add the feta, a squeeze of lemon juice, and a drizzle of oil. Add a pinch or two of sumac and a pinch of salt, then serve.

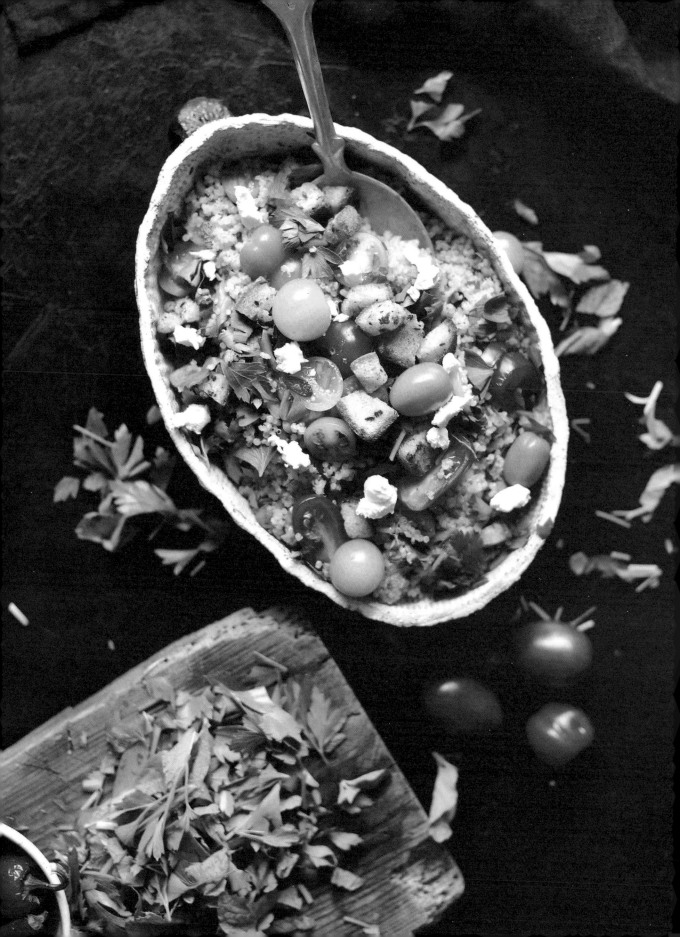

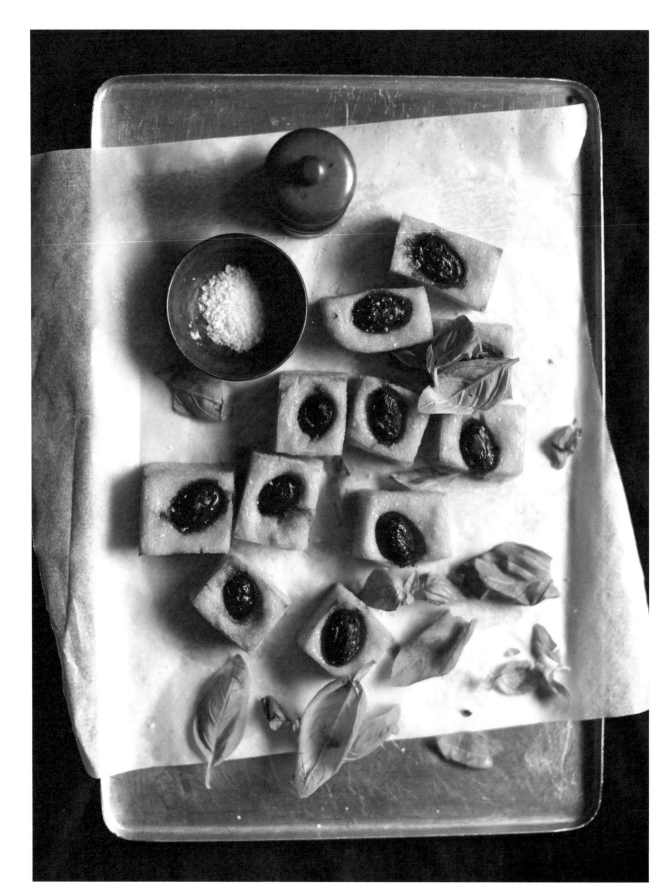

Olive and Parmesan Polenta Squares

SERVES 6
as a starter

When you've ticked the "vegetarian" box at functions for as long as you can remember, it's difficult not to associate polenta with those hard, flavorless slabs of yellow that get dropped in front of you after the salad starter and before the risotto main. The key to polenta, I've discovered, is cooking it in stock instead of water—that, and beating in lots of grated cheese, which is really the answer to most things.

Butter, for greasing and frying
4 cups (1 L) FODMAP-friendly vegetable stock (such as My Go-To Veggie Stock, page 62)
1 cup (180 g) instant polenta
1 cup (100 g) freshly grated vegetarian Parmesan
Zest of ½ lemon
½ teaspoon sea salt
⅔ cup (100 g) pitted kalamata olives

1. Lightly grease a 7 × 11-inch (18 × 28 cm) brownie pan or baking dish with butter. In a large saucepan, combine the stock and polenta and cook over medium-high heat for 5 to 10 minutes. Stir continuously, until it thickens and bubbles.

2. Remove from the heat and stir in the Parmesan, lemon zest, and salt. Pour into the greased pan and gently press the olives into the polenta. Set aside for 10 to 15 minutes to set.

3. Once the polenta has set, carefully turn it out onto a chopping board and slice into portions. Heat a knob of butter in a medium frying pan over medium-high heat. Fry the slices of polenta until golden, and then serve by themselves, or as a side.

My Go-To Veggie Stock

MAKES
4 QUARTS (4 L)

It has taken me many years to realize that stock shouldn't, and needn't, come in a solid block. Not only is it easy to make, but it's super customizable and a really simple way to add flavor to things that might otherwise be average (prime examples being the Quinoa, Fresh Tomato, and Fried Bread Salad on page 58 or the Crispy Sage Breakfast Hash on page 29). I use fennel in my stock because cooked celery makes me recoil (and, conveniently for me, it's only FODMAP-friendly in servings of a quarter of a stick or less). I would never condone celery use, but you can play around and use whatever works for you personally.

2½ tablespoons olive oil

3 large carrots, roughly chopped

2 fennel bulbs, quartered

7 ounces (200 g) cremini mushrooms or other strong-flavored mushrooms of your choice

⅓ cup (80 ml) gluten-free tamari

2 to 3 teaspoons sea salt

1. Place the oil and carrot in your largest stockpot and begin to sweat them off over medium-high heat.
2. After a few minutes, add the fennel and mushrooms, followed by the tamari.
3. Add a little splash of the water to the pot now if the veggies are starting to stick. Continue cooking until the vegetables are golden and have softened, then add 4 quarts (4 L) water and the salt.
4. Bring the stock to a boil and then turn the heat down to a gentle simmer. Cook for at least 20 minutes before straining and discarding the vegetables. You can store this in the fridge for a few days in an airtight container, or freeze it in smaller batches, so it's ready to go whenever you need it.

Peanut, Makrut Lime, and Squash Soup

SERVES 2

If there were an opportunity to door knock and extol the virtues of makrut lime, I would undoubtedly volunteer (does repeating myself in a cookbook count?). Makrut lime is my favorite way to add an exotic flavor to Southeast Asian–inspired dishes, without the need for shallots or onion. A grating of makrut lime zest, if you can find it, is the star of this soup, which just happens to be FODMAP friendly and vegan.

2½ tablespoons peanut oil

10 makrut lime leaves (see Note)

1-inch (3 cm) piece fresh ginger, finely sliced

1 lemongrass stem, bruised

1 teaspoon finely grated makrut lime zest

2½ tablespoons FODMAP-Friendly Kecap Manis (page 81)

2½ tablespoons gluten-free tamari

5 cups (700 g) peeled, diced kabocha squash

2 cups (500 ml) FODMAP-friendly vegetable stock (such as My Go-To-Veggie Stock, page 62)

1 cup plus 2 tablespoons (270 ml) coconut milk (make sure it doesn't contain inulin)

⅓ cup (90 g) smooth natural peanut butter, plus extra to serve

1 to 2 teaspoons hot sauce, or to taste (make sure it doesn't contain garlic or onion)

To serve

Coconut yogurt

Cilantro leaves

Fresh red chile, finely sliced (optional)

1. In a large saucepan, heat the oil and add the lime leaves, ginger, lemongrass, and lime zest. Cook over medium heat—they should become fragrant within a minute or two.

2. Add the kecap manis, tamari, and squash and stir intermittently until the squash is coated and beginning to sweat. Add the stock, turn up the heat, and cook for around 20 minutes, until the squash is soft.

3. Remove from the heat and add the coconut milk, peanut butter, and hot sauce. Using an immersion blender or food processor (be very careful when blitzing really hot liquid in the processor—it's best to let the soup cool if you are going this route), blend the soup to a smooth consistency.

4. Serve with a dollop of coconut yogurt, another little spoonful of peanut butter, a few cilantro leaves, and chile slices, if using, scattered on top.

Note: I buy makrut lime leaves in the frozen section of my local Asian grocer, although I've noticed them popping up in fresh form at my local supermarket. Makrut limes are harder to find—they are seasonal and often found in the freezer section. When they're available, I buy them in bulk and keep them in my freezer, and I grate the zest into curries and satay and onto tofu.

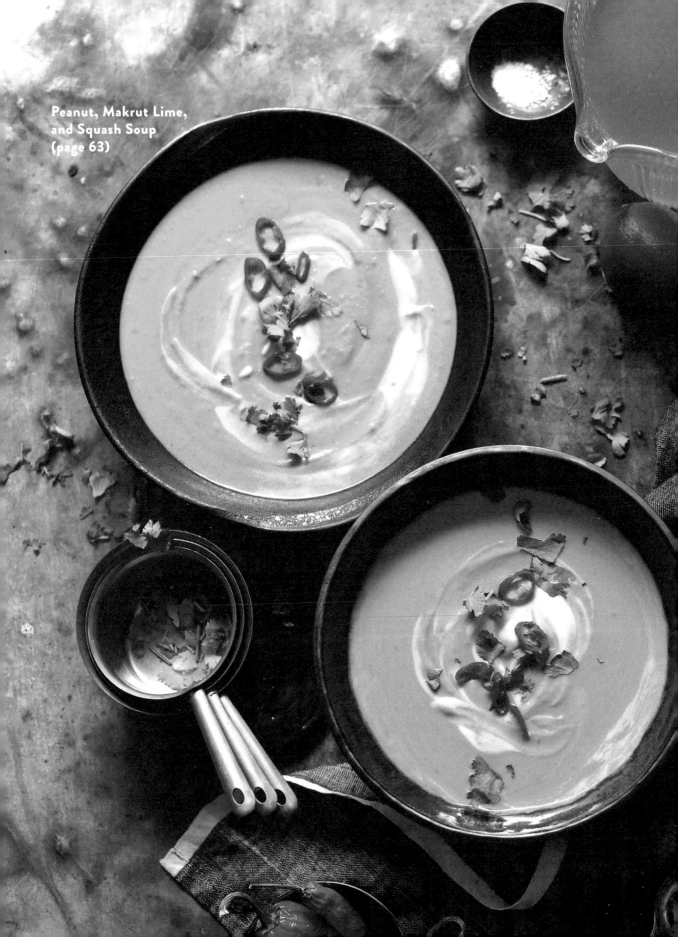

Peanut, Makrut Lime,
and Squash Soup
(page 63)

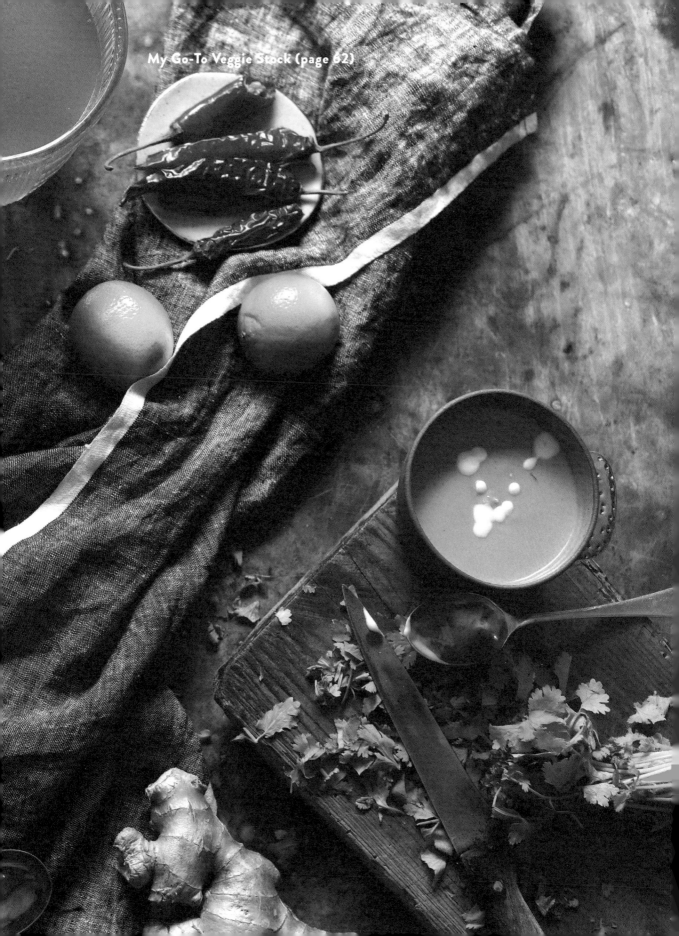

My Go-To Veggie Stock (page 62)

Vegetarian Pho

Vietnam is one of my all-time favorite travel destinations, and at least 70 percent of that assessment is a direct result of the national dish, pho. While pho is traditionally made with a beef broth heavy in onion and garlic, I've created an inadvertently vegan and advertently FODMAP-friendly version. Shiitake mushrooms add a necessary depth to the broth, but you can adjust the amount if they are a trigger for you.

Pho broth

4 cinnamon sticks
7 star anise
2 cloves
1 tablespoon peanut or sesame oil
2 large carrots, roughly chopped
1 large fennel bulb, roughly chopped (you can throw the fronds in, too)
1-inch (3 cm) piece fresh ginger, finely sliced
1 cup (75 g) sliced fresh shiitake mushrooms
⅓ cup (80 ml) gluten-free tamari, plus extra for the tofu
1 bunch Thai basil or cilantro, leaves picked, stems discarded
1 bunch Vietnamese mint or other mint, leaves picked, stems discarded

To serve

7 ounces (200 g) firm tofu, cubed or sliced
1 large carrot, julienned
1 bunch bok choy, chopped if large
9 ounces (250 g) rice noodles
Fresh red chile, finely sliced
Lime wedges

1. **To make the broth,** place a large saucepan over medium heat and dry-fry the cinnamon, star anise, and cloves for a minute or two, until fragrant. Add the oil, carrot, and fennel and cook for a couple of minutes until it begins to sizzle. Add the ginger, shiitakes, and a splash of water and continue to cook for another couple of minutes.

2. Add the tamari and cook until once it has reduced down and caramelized on the bottom of the pan, then add the water. Cover and bring the broth to a boil. Add a handful of the herbs, reduce to medium heat, and cook for 20 minutes.

3. **Meanwhile, to finish,** dry-fry the tofu in a medium frying pan over a medium heat, until it starts to crisp up, 3 to 5 minutes, and then pour over a splash of tamari. Remove the pan from the heat and transfer to a plate, then rinse out the frying pan and return it to the heat. Gently cook the carrots with a splash of water for 5 minutes, then add the bok choy and cook for 5 more minutes, until tender. Remove from the heat.

4. Prepare the rice noodles per package instructions.

5. To assemble, divide the noodles between four serving bowls and then arrange the tofu, carrot, and bok choy on top. Ladle in the pho broth and finish the bowls with some fresh chile, the remaining herbs, and wedges of lime.

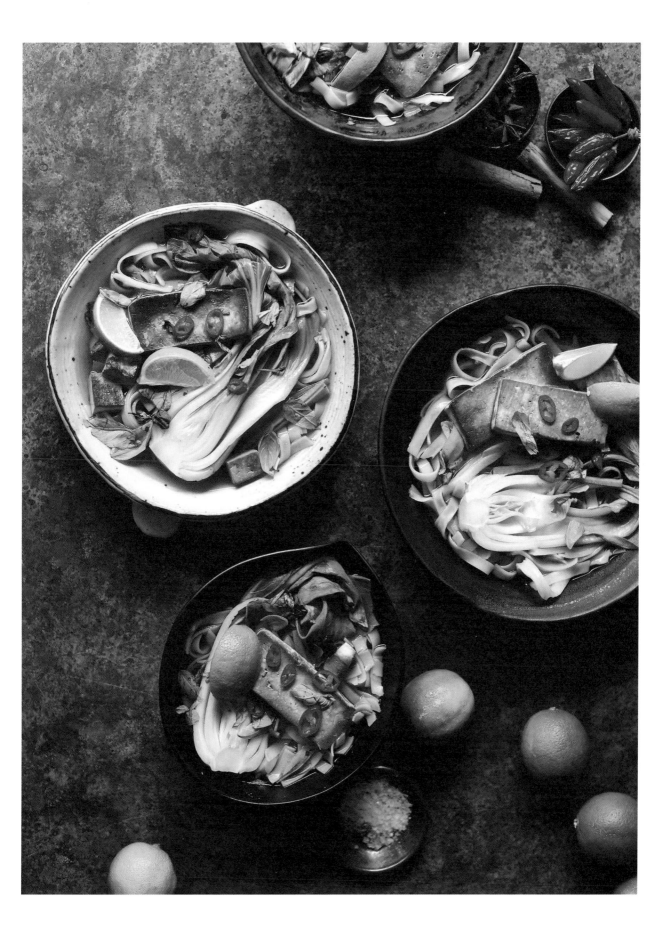

Vegetarian Nachos

I mean, are you really going to make me introduce nachos? These are the full package: vegetarian taco "meat," a FODMAP-friendly queso, and FODMAP-friendly guacamole. My deep dive into queso tells me that there is a certain brand of tomatoes associated with the delicacy, and that Monterey Jack is a cheese of choice. I couldn't find either of those in Australia, but Gouda, Gruyère, and Swiss are all worthy substitutes.

Chili

16 ounces (450 g) tofu, frozen
¼ cup (60 ml) olive oil
1 fennel bulb, finely chopped
1 medium carrot, chopped
1 jalapeño, seeded and chopped
1 poblano chile, seeded and chopped
1 tablespoon cumin seeds
1 tablespoon ground cumin
1 tablespoon smoked paprika
1 teaspoon cinnamon
Generous cracked black pepper
2½ tablespoons tomato paste
One 28-ounce (794 g) can diced tomatoes, with green chiles (preferably Ro-Tel)
1 tablespoon gluten-free miso
2 to 4 teaspoons gluten-free tamari
2½ tablespoons lime juice
1 tablespoon light brown sugar
1 to 2 ounces (25 to 50 g) baking chocolate (70 percent cocoa) or 2 teaspoons cocoa powder
½ cup (125 ml) FODMAP-friendly vegetable stock (such as My Go-To Veggie Stock, page 62) or water

Queso

2½ tablespoons (40 g) butter
4 jalapeños, seeded and chopped
1 teaspoon light brown sugar
1 teaspoon cumin
1 teaspoon smoked paprika
1 teaspoon white vinegar
2 large tomatoes, chopped
2½ tablespoons gluten-free cornstarch
¾ to 1 cup (180 to 250 ml) lactose-free milk, depending on how thick you like your dip
2 cups (200 g) grated Monterey Jack cheese
1½ cups (150 g) grated sharp cheddar

1. **To make the chili,** defrost the tofu using your preferred method. I like to heat it in a heatproof sieve over a pot of water, double boiler style. Squeeze out the excess liquid and set aside.

2. Warm a heavy-bottomed saucepan over medium heat, then add the oil. Add the fennel, carrot, jalapeño, poblano, and spices and cook until they begin to brown and soften, 10 to 15 minutes. If they start to stick to the pan, lower the heat and add a splash of water.

3. Add the canned tomatoes and stir well to combine. Cook for a few minutes before adding the remaining ingredients, one at a time. Stir after each addition.

4. Crumble the tofu into the mixture, creating small pieces resembling ground meat. Stir well and cook for 15 to 20 minutes. Add extra stock or water if you prefer a thinner chili.

5. **To make the queso,** melt the butter in a medium-large pot over medium heat, then add the jalapeños, sugar, cumin, paprika, and vinegar. Stir and cook for 5 to 10 minutes, until the jalapeños soften.

6. Add the tomatoes and cook for 5 to 10 minutes, until the liquid thickens and appears yellow-orange.

7. Whisk in the cornstarch and cook for 10 seconds or so, whisking constantly. Add the milk, whisk to combine, and cook until thickened.

8. Gently whisk in the grated cheese until a smooth sauce forms.

9. **To finish,** arrange the chips in a baking dish and top with as much of the chili and queso as you'd like. Broil in the oven for 15 to 20 minutes.

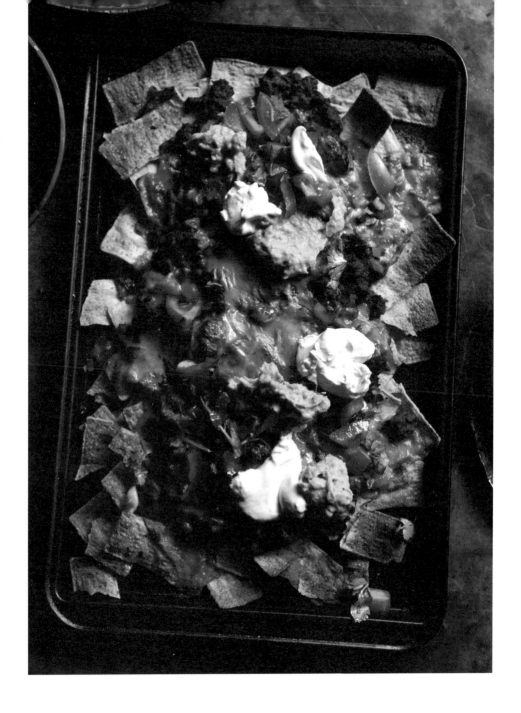

To finish

1 large bag tortilla chips
1 to 2 avocados
Lime juice
Sea salt flakes
1 to 2 large fresh tomatoes,
   chopped
Cilantro, chopped
Sour cream

10. Meanwhile, mash the avocado with some lime juice and salt in a small bowl. Combine the tomatoes with some cilantro, lime juice, and salt in another bowl.

11. Remove the nachos from the oven, then add the avocado, sour cream, and tomato salsa. Serve immediately.

Tempeh Nut Falafels

MAKES ABOUT 20
SMALL FALAFELS
(enough for 6 people
as a side dish)

I'm with you—tempeh is a terrifying-looking ingredient for the uninitiated (and sometimes for the initiated as well). That said, falafels are traditionally made with high-FODMAP chickpeas, so tempeh is the closest FODMAP-friendly legume product we've got. These go well with Coconut Flatbreads (page 111).

1 cup (150 g) sunflower seeds
10 ounces (300 g) unflavored
   tempeh
1 tablespoon ground cumin
1 teaspoon red pepper flakes
1 teaspoon allspice
Pinch of ground nutmeg
1 teaspoon sea salt
1 large piece (30 g) preserved
   lemon rind, finely chopped
¾ cup (20 g) mint leaves, plus
   extra to garnish
¾ cup (20 g) cilantro leaves, plus
   extra to garnish
⅓ cup (80 ml) olive oil

To serve
Coconut and Cucumber Tzatziki
   (page 71)

1. Preheat the oven to 350°F (180°C). Line a baking sheet with parchment paper.
2. Pulse the sunflower seeds in a food processor to create a fine sunflower seed meal. Add the rest of the ingredients and process until completely combined. If the mixture is really thick and dry, add a small splash of water to make it a little easier to work with.
3. Use your hands to create about twenty small balls. Place these on the lined baking sheet as you make them.
4. Bake the falafels for 10 to 15 minutes, until lightly browned on top, and then turn them over. Return to the oven and bake for another 10 to 15 minutes until they are golden.
5. Serve with the tzatziki and extra herbs.

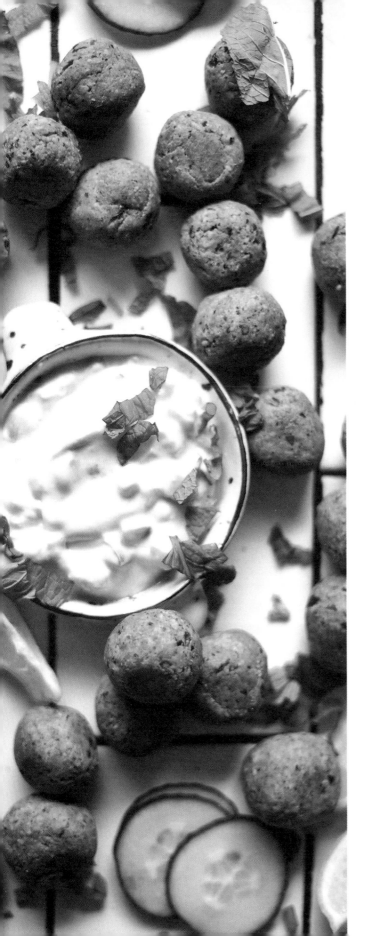

Coconut and Cucumber Tzatziki

This is a simple alternative for the regular tzatziki we all know and love. It's dairy-free and garlic-free, but it gets a bit of a kick thanks to the preserved lemon juice.

¾ cup (150 g) plain coconut yogurt
¾ cup (100 g) chopped cucumber
2 teaspoons preserved lemon brine (the juices in your jar of preserved lemon)
1 tablespoon fresh lemon or lime juice
1 tablespoon chopped mint, to garnish (optional)

1. Mix the yogurt, cucumber, lemon brine, and lemon juice together.
2. Allow to stand for a couple of hours in the fridge before serving for the best flavor. Garnish with the mint, if using.

Salt and Vinegar Smashed Roasted Potatoes

SERVES 4 TO 6
as a side dish

Although there's no such thing as getting tired of potatoes, these magnificent creatures are here to spruce up your potato repertoire. By boiling the potatoes in vinegar prior to baking them, their flesh is pierced with a delicious vinegar tang before their edges are crisped in the oven. Like salt and vinegar chips, only ten times better. I like to serve these with mixed herbs and some arugula, but I also like them with a big bowl of Kewpie mayo and not much else.

2 pounds (1 kg) baby potatoes for roasting (I used Kipfler here, but creamer potatoes such as Yukon Gold and new potatoes will work well)

4 to 5 cups (1 to 1.2 L) white vinegar (I buy a 2 L bottle to make sure I have enough to cover the potatoes)

Generous good-quality sea salt flakes

Generous good-quality olive oil, to cover the bottom of a large baking sheet

Knob of butter (optional)

1. Generously prick each potato with a fork (about eight to ten fork pricks should do it—this is to allow the vinegar to permeate the potato).

2. Place them in a medium pot and cover with the vinegar and a sprinkle of sea salt. Turn the heat to medium high and allow the potatoes to bubble away for a good 15 to 20 minutes, until they are easily poked with a knife. Turn the heat off and allow them to sit in the vinegar for 5 minutes or so.

3. Preheat the oven to 350°F (180°C). Drain the potatoes in a colander and allow them to steam dry and cool a little, for 10 to 15 minutes.

4. While the potatoes are cooling, coat the bottom of a large baking sheet with the oil and place it into the oven. If you're using the butter, add that, too.

5. Once the potatoes have cooled a bit, use your hand or a potato ricer to roughly smash them. The more edges exposed, the more crispiness! Sprinkle some more salt into the hot oil, and follow this with the smashed potatoes. They should sizzle a little on impact, which will start forming a crispy base straight off the bat.

6. Now for some patience. For maximum crunchiness, cook the potatoes for at least an hour, if not an hour and 20 minutes, flipping halfway through. You can take them out whenever you need to, but the crunchiness is worth waiting for, if you have the time.

7. Sprinkle with a little more salt and serve with whatever you fancy.

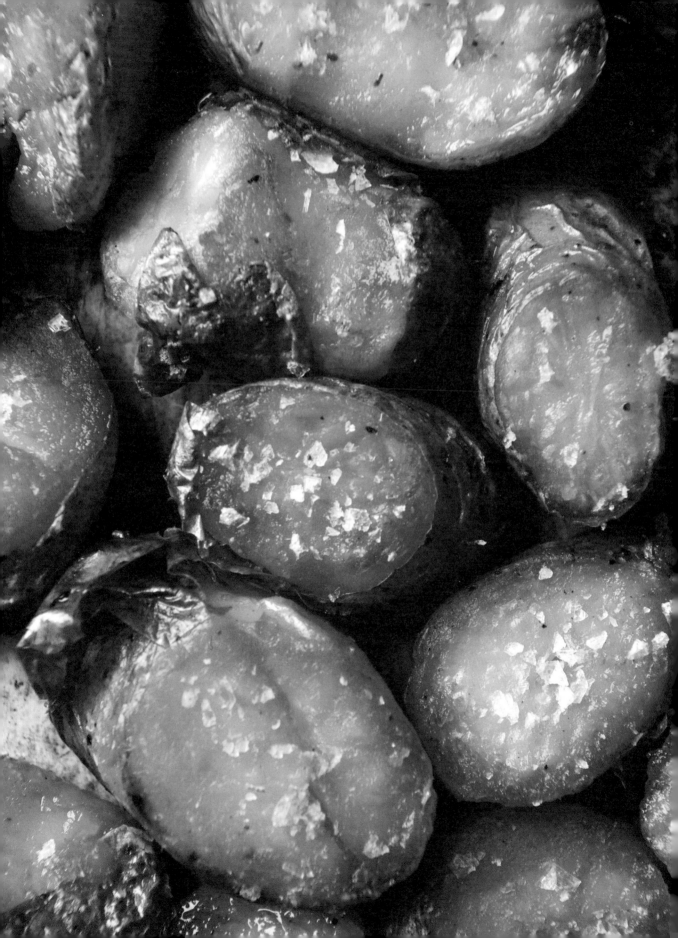

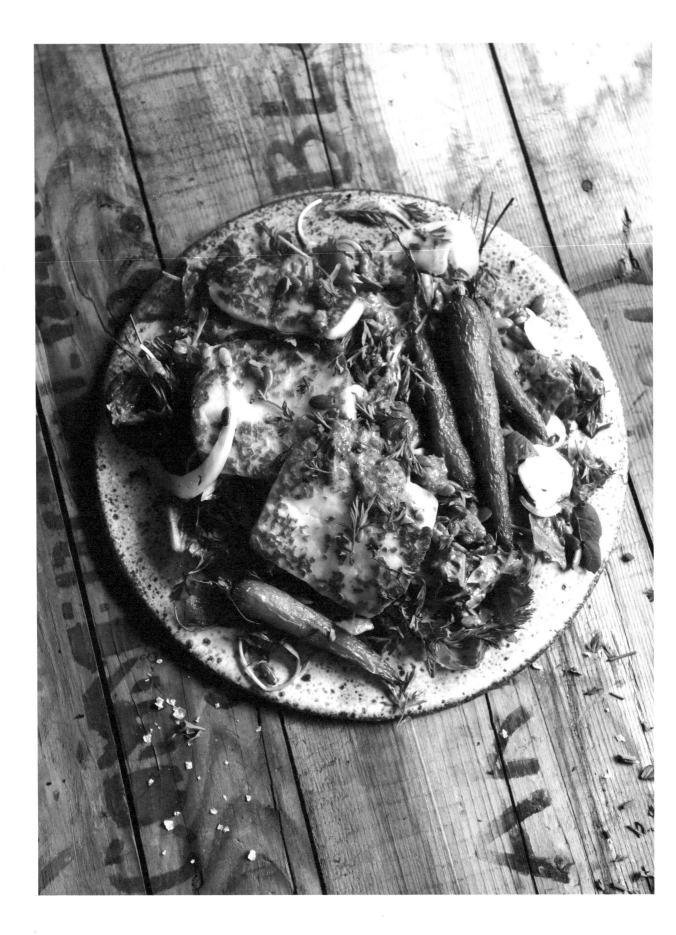

Honey Butter Roasted Carrot and Halloumi Salad

SERVES 4 TO 6
as a side dish

Strangers regularly tag me in photos of halloumi on Instagram, thanks to my aggressive pursuit of halloumi-based recipes in the earlier days of my online career. This recipe is one of my halloumi-related standouts, if such a thing could even exist.

Honey butter roasted carrots

9 ounces (250 g) small carrots, washed and trimmed

1 to 2 tablespoons (15–30 g) butter (if you use more, you can drizzle the extra mixture over the salad at the end, heyo!)

1 teaspoon honey

Herb and lemon dressing

1 large bunch mint

1 large bunch cilantro

½ cup (125 ml) good-quality olive oil

1 large piece (30 g) preserved lemon (the whole thing, not just the flesh)

Juice of 1 lemon

Good pinch of sea salt

Massaged fennel

1 fennel bulb, thinly sliced

1 tablespoon olive oil

Lemon juice, to taste

Sea salt, to taste

Sea salt pepitas

½ cup (80 g) pepitas

2 teaspoons maple syrup or honey

1 teaspoon sea salt

To finish

Neutral oil, for frying

1 packet of halloumi (these vary in weight, but just buy the bigger one, amirite)

2 large handfuls greens of choice (sprouts, carrot tops, lettuce, arugula, and microgreens all work well)

1. Preheat the oven to 350°F (180°C). Line a baking sheet with parchment paper.
2. To make the carrots, place them on another sheet of parchment paper. Dot with small pieces of the butter (I use my hands) and the honey (I do not use my hands). Roast in the oven for 30 minutes to 1 hour, depending on the size of your carrots and how "done" you like them. I cook mine for an hour, because I like them well cooked and the honey caramelized.
3. Meanwhile, to make the dressing, combine all the ingredients and blend until a smooth sauce forms. Set aside.
4. To make the fennel, place it in a large bowl and massage in the oil and lemon juice with your hands. Sprinkle with salt and allow to sit.
5. To make the pepitas, when the carrots have about 10 minutes left, spread the pepitas on the prepared baking sheet. Bake for 10 minutes or until browned, remove from the oven, and drizzle with the maple syrup and salt, mixing well.
6. To finish, pull the carrots out of the oven. Heat a little oil in a nonstick frying pan over high heat and cook the halloumi, until soft and golden on both sides. Remove from the heat.
7. Place the greens on a serving plate and top with the fennel, carrots, pepitas, halloumi, and the dressing.

Miso Maple Greens

This recipe makes me sound like I have my life together infinitely more than I do, but I love having a batch of these greens in the fridge, ready for when hunger strikes (roughly every ten minutes at my house). They're perfect as a side with some protein, as a snack on their own, or thrown in with some scrambled eggs. You can play around with any FODMAP-friendly vegetables that take your fancy.

About 2 pounds (1 kg) zucchini and broccoli, or other mix of low-FODMAP green vegetables

Miso dressing

1 tablespoon gluten-free miso
1 tablespoon maple syrup
1 tablespoon boiling water
2 teaspoons apple cider vinegar
2 teaspoons toasted sesame oil
Hot sauce, to taste

To serve

Large handful baby spinach

1. Preheat the oven to 350°F (180°C). Line a baking sheet or roasting pan with parchment paper.
2. Spread the vegetables evenly across the baking sheet and place in the oven for 20 minutes, or until the zucchini is soft and the broccoli is crispy.
3. To make the miso dressing, place the ingredients in a small bowl and whisk until thoroughly combined.
4. To serve, remove the cooked vegetables from the oven and toss them into a large bowl with the spinach. Pour the miso dressing on top and stir gently to coat. Serve warm or store for later. These keep well in the fridge for a few days in an airtight container.

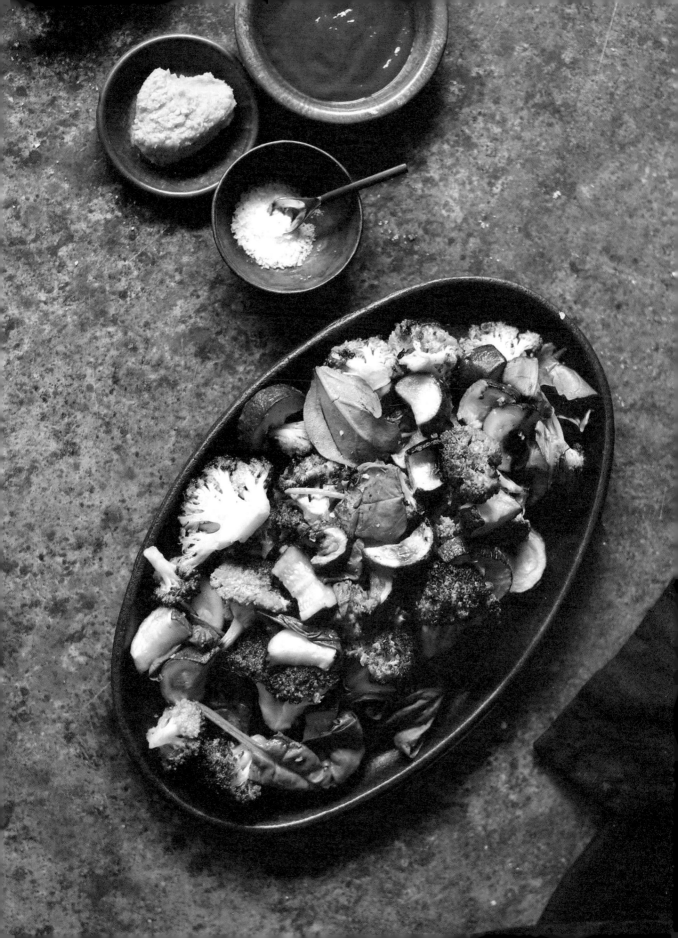

Orange, Olive, and Dill Salad with Star Anise Dressing

This punchy number is my ideal hot-weather salad—something to replace the classic watermelon, feta, and olive number. It's a great balance of salty and sweet, with added depth from the star anise dressing. The flavors come together even more overnight, so it makes for great leftovers the next day. A thinly sliced cucumber or two can be added to round out the salad.

Star anise dressing

2½ tablespoons olive oil

2½ tablespoons freshly squeezed lemon or lime juice

4 star anise

1 teaspoon maple syrup

Salad

4 oranges

⅓ cup (50 g) pitted kalamata olives, halved

Handful of dill, chopped

⅓ cup (50 g) crumbled feta

1. To make the dressing, combine all of the ingredients in a small saucepan and place over medium-high heat until bubbling. Turn the heat down slightly, stir intermittently, and cook for an additional 5 minutes so it thickens and reduces. Set aside to cool a little.

2. To assemble the salad, peel and slice the oranges and arrange them on a serving plate. Scatter the olives, dill, and feta on top. Drizzle with the warm star anise dressing and serve.

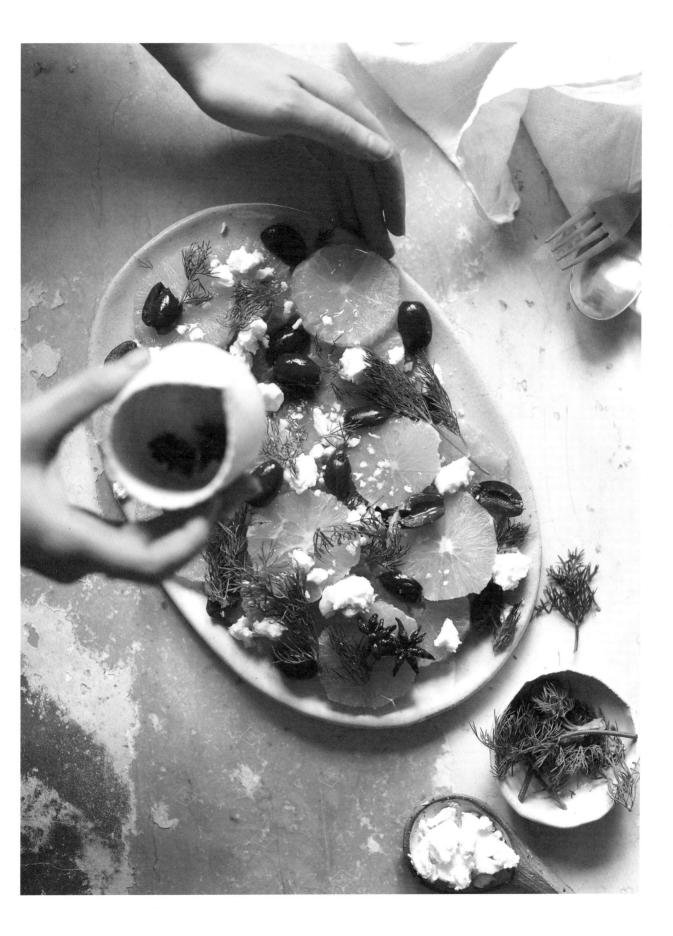

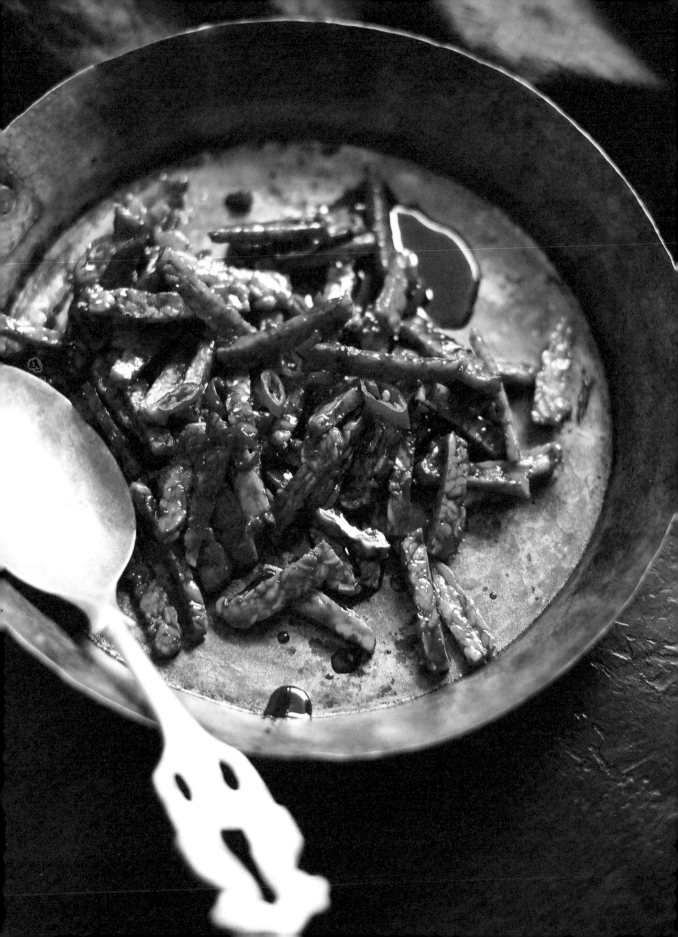

Kecap Tempeh

I first tried kecap tempeh on a trip to Bali in my early twenties, and it was a true revelation. The crunchy fried tempeh is coated in a sticky, sweet, makrut lime–perfumed sauce and then dotted with pieces of fresh chile. You can eat it alone, as I often do (in more ways than one), or with rice and Asian greens, or use it as a salad-sprucing protein.

FODMAP-Friendly Kecap Manis

2½ tablespoons maple syrup

¼ cup (60 ml) gluten-free tamari

Tempeh

8 ounces (225 g) tempeh

¼ to ⅓ cup (60 to 80 ml) peanut oil

2 teaspoons coconut sugar (optional)

1 to 2 teaspoons finely grated fresh ginger

Zest of ½ makrut lime (or 3 to 4 makrut lime leaves, finely sliced)

1. To make the kecap manis, combine the maple syrup and tamari in a small saucepan over medium heat. Cook, stirring intermittently, until it begins to bubble and thicken. Remove from the heat and leave to cool. Done!

2. To make the tempeh, cut the tempeh into reasonably thin slices (about 5 mm) and then into matchsticks.

3. Heat the oil in a large frying pan over high heat and fry the tempeh until crunchy and golden. Transfer to a plate lined with paper towels and allow to drain.

4. Pour out most of the oil from the pan, then return to the heat. Pour in the kecap manis and add the sugar (if using), ginger, and lime zest. Cook for 2 to 3 minutes, until the sugar has melted and the mixture is fragrant.

5. Return the tempeh to the pan and toss to coat evenly in the sticky sauce. Serve hot.

Makrut Lime Satay Tofu with Vietnamese-Style Coleslaw

SERVES 4
as an appetizer or
2 as a main

In case you haven't noticed yet, I am in a committed relationship with makrut lime. The zest makes the tastiest satay, but if you can't find the fruit itself, substitute with five or six large makrut lime leaves and a small handful of Thai basil and Vietnamese mint leaves (just remember to take them out of the sauce before serving). I buy my makrut limes and leaves from Asian grocers, and they're most often found in the freezer section.

Makrut lime satay sauce

1 tablespoon peanut oil
1 teaspoon finely grated makrut lime zest
1 tablespoon gluten-free tamari
2 teaspoons FODMAP-Friendly Kecap Manis (page 81)
1 teaspoon hot sauce, plus extra to taste
½ cup (140 g) peanut butter
1 cup (250 ml) boiling water

Tofu

2 teaspoons tapioca flour
7 ounces (200 g) firm tofu, drained

Coleslaw

2 cups (150 g) finely sliced cabbage, a mixture of red and white is nice
Handful of Thai basil (or cilantro) and Vietnamese (or other) mint, finely sliced, plus extra to garnish
1 cup (100 g) julienned carrots
1 cup (100 g) finely sliced cucumber
1 tablespoon rice wine vinegar
1 tablespoon FODMAP-Friendly Kecap Manis
1 teaspoon gluten-free tamari
½ a juicy lime
2 teaspoons coconut sugar

1. Preheat the oven to 350°F (180°C). Line a baking sheet with parchment paper.
2. To make the satay sauce, heat the oil in a large frying pan over medium heat, then add the lime zest, tamari, kecap manis, and hot sauce. Allow to bubble for a minute or so.
3. Gently stir in the peanut butter, then pour in the boiling water. Continue to stir until the mixture thickens, 2 to 3 minutes.
4. Remove from the heat, transfer to a wide shallow bowl, and leave to cool.
5. To make the tofu, pour the tapioca flour into a wide shallow bowl. Cut the tofu into cubes and, working in batches, lightly coat them in the tapioca flour. Carefully dip the tofu in the satay sauce to completely coat each piece, then transfer to the lined baking sheet.
6. Bake the tofu in the oven for about 20 minutes, until crunchy and golden. Set aside.
7. To make the coleslaw, combine the cabbage and herbs in a large bowl, then add the carrot and cucumber. Mix the remaining ingredients together in a small bowl, then massage this dressing into the coleslaw with your hands.
8. To serve, divide the coleslaw between plates, top with the tofu and extra herbs, and serve right away.

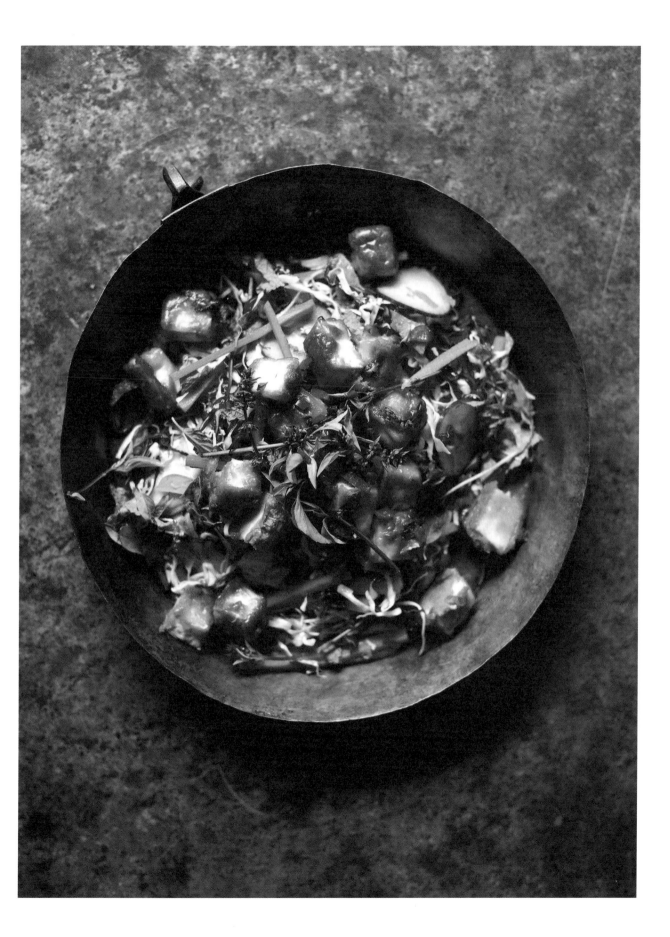

Vegetarian Caesar Salad with Salt and Pepper Tofu Croutons

SERVES 4

This is what happens when you let the vegetarians have free rein: They go ahead and make all the classics better. Just kidding (kind of). This Caesar salad uses crispy salt and pepper tofu in place of croutons to make it a more substantial meal. Of course, if you were to add croutons as well, you'd receive nothing but praise from me. I prefer to use vegan mayonnaise here, because I unashamedly prefer the taste. You can use whatever you'd prefer. To make this entirely vegan, simply use vegan substitutes for the mayonnaise and Parmesan, and omit the eggs.

Caesar dressing

1 cup (230 g) mayo
½ cup (50 g) finely grated vegetarian
  Parmesan, plus extra slices to serve
2 to 2½ tablespoons lemon juice
1 teaspoon mustard
2 teaspoons FODMAP-Friendly Vegan
  Worcestershire Sauce (page 86)
2 teaspoons finely chopped capers
1 teaspoon caper brine
Freshly cracked black pepper
Plant-based milk (optional)

Salt and pepper tofu croutons

16 ounces (450 g) firm tofu, drained
  and pressed (see Note on page 119)
2½ tablespoons gluten-free cornstarch
½ teaspoon fine salt
Lots of freshly cracked black pepper
Neutral oil, for frying (vegetable,
  canola, or peanut are good, but
  peanut will add nuts)

Salad

2 large heads romaine lettuce or 1
  head radicchio, chopped if leaves
  are large
Arugula (optional)
Finely chopped flat-leaf parsley
  (optional)
4 soft-boiled eggs, halved
More freshly cracked black pepper
Sea salt flakes

1. To make the dressing, mix all the ingredients together and set aside. Taste and adjust for seasoning (the more pepper, the better). Use some milk to thin it out, if desired.

2. To make the salt and pepper tofu croutons, combine the cornstarch, salt, and pepper in a large bowl. Tear the tofu into the bowl in bite-size crouton-style chunks. (Tearing it, as opposed to cutting it, gives it nice craggy edges that become crispy. You can do half torn and half cut if you prefer.) Toss with your hands to thoroughly coat.

3. Heat a large heavy-bottomed pan with some oil over medium-high heat. Add the tofu in batches, cooking for a couple minutes on all sides and until golden brown. Transfer to a plate lined with paper towels and repeat until all the tofu is done.

4. Depending on the brand you've chosen, you might have some crumbly tofu bits leftover. Cook them at the end—they add delicious little chunks of crunchiness.

5. To assemble the salad, arrange the lettuce on a plate and top with the tofu croutons, the arugula and parsley, if using, and the dressing. You can toss to coat, if that's your thing. Finish with the eggs, sliced in half, some extra slices of Parmesan, a crack of pepper, and some salt. This keeps well in the fridge for a few days.

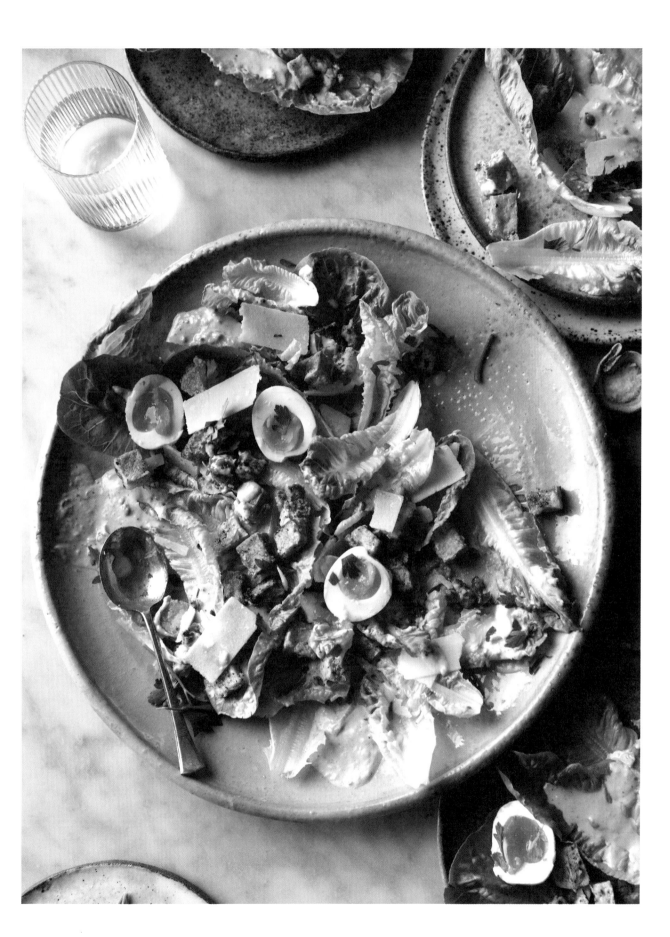

FODMAP-Friendly Vegan Worcestershire Sauce

MAKES ABOUT
⅓ CUP (80 ML)

Regular Worcestershire sauce contains anchovies, onion, and garlic. There are some vegetarian varieties on the market, and the onion and garlic should present no issue in such a small quantity. However, if you'd like to make your own, this recipe has none of the above.

½ cup (120 ml) apple cider vinegar

2½ tablespoons gluten-free tamari

2½ tablespoons light brown sugar

1 teaspoon maple syrup

½ teaspoon ground cinnamon

½ teaspoon ground allspice

Pinch of ground clove (optional)

Freshly cracked black pepper

1. Combine the vinegar, tamari, sugar, maple syrup, cinnamon, allspice, and clove, if using, in a small saucepan over medium heat. Stir intermittently for 10 to 15 minutes, until the sauce has thickened.

2. Add some pepper, and use in whatever you're doing (Vegan Bolognese, page 93, obviously encouraged). Store in an airtight container and use within a week or two.

Pumpkin Curry

SERVES 4

Think of this recipe as your FODMAP-friendly, not-rubbish equivalent to a jar of curry sauce. The pumpkin lends a sweetness to the sauce, effectively removing the need for onion. You can add whatever else you'd normally add to your curry, but I've included my go-to ingredients below. Enjoy this as is or with rice.

4⅓ cups (500 g) peeled and cubed pumpkin or other winter squash, cut into 1-inch (2.5 cm) pieces

¼ cup (60 ml) plus 1 tablespoon vegetable oil

1 tablespoon garam masala

2 teaspoons ground cumin

1 teaspoon ground turmeric

½ teaspoon ground cinnamon

1 to 2 teaspoons finely grated fresh ginger

1 cup (250 ml) coconut milk (make sure it doesn't contain inulin)

8 ounces (225 g) tempeh, diced (see Note)

1 pound (500 g) vegetables of your choice, roughly chopped (I like to use zucchini and bok choy)

Fresh chile, finely chopped, to taste

1. Using your preferred method, steam the pumpkin cubes until soft and well cooked. Set aside.
2. In a large frying pan, heat the ¼ cup (60 ml) oil over medium heat and, once warmed, add the spices. Cook for a minute or so until aromatic, and then add the ginger.
3. Add the steamed pumpkin to the pan and continue cooking for a few minutes, until the pumpkin is well coated in spices and completely softened.
4. Transfer the pumpkin mixture into a food processor (make sure you get all the spices). Allow it to cool for a few minutes (so it doesn't explode on you) and then blitz until the mixture is completely smooth.
5. Return the frying pan to the heat and add the remaining tablespoon oil. Return the pumpkin mixture to the pan, add the coconut milk, and stir thoroughly. Add the tempeh and your vegetables of choice, and cook until the vegetables are soft.
6. Serve with some chile sprinkled on top.

Note: You can save some of the diced tempeh to use as a garnish if you like. Fry it lightly in oil until nice and crispy, then sprinkle on top for a little crunch.

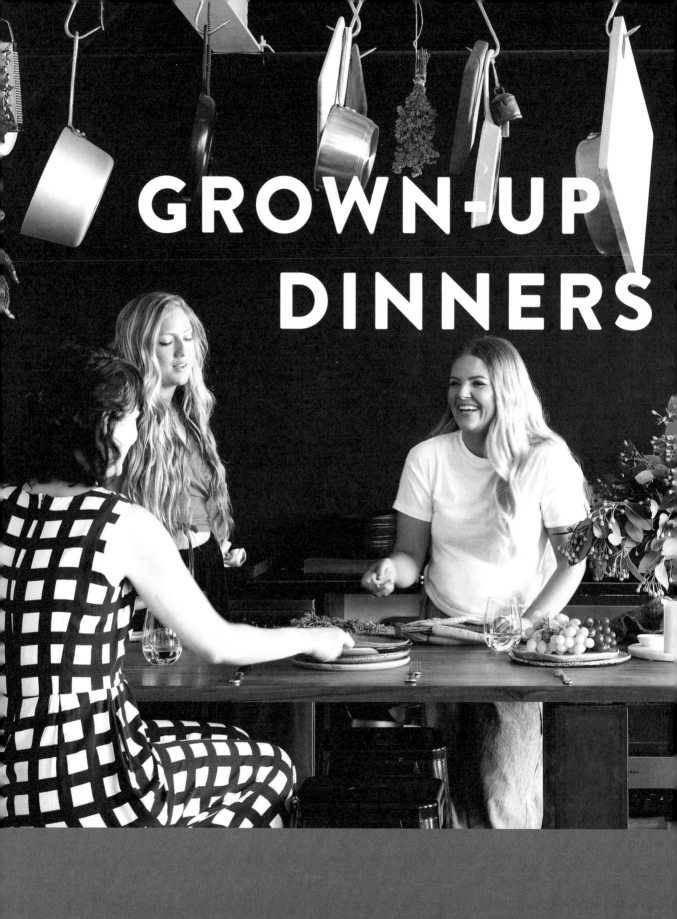

GROWN-UP DINNERS

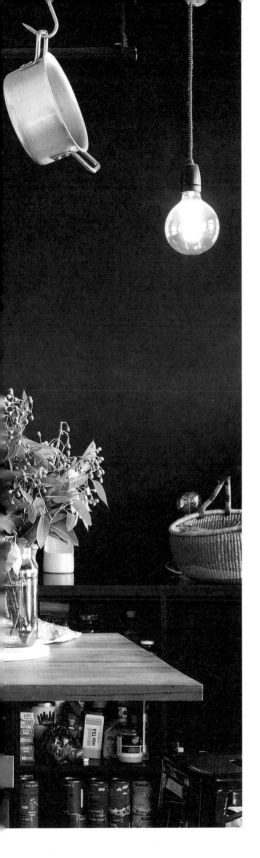

Can you tell this chapter was named by someone who has spent much of their twenties eating cheese on cucumber for dinner?

Acquiring dinner that doesn't contain onion, garlic, gluten, or a combination of the above has generally proven a challenge for me. I'd prefer not to comment on how many times I've said, "I can eat the salad," when skimming a menu or a barbecue table.

This chapter is filled with some of my favorite adult recipes, from shahi paneer to vegan laksa. I wanted to create a resource for people dealing with digestive illnesses but also for their friends, families, and significant others. Because nobody should have to pretend to be excited about eating salad as a main course (unless they want to).

So, yes, some of the recipes are a little more labor-intensive than cheese on cucumber. If you've reached peak adult status, however, you might have some room for freezing leftovers. You know, among the hangover ice pops and frozen banana graveyard you're "saving for banana bread."

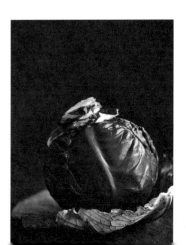

Vegan Potato Gnocchi

SERVES 6 TO 8

Your new hero for hosting a dietary-niche dinner party is this five-ingredient vegan *and* gluten-free gnocchi—it uses naught but readily available flours and the magic of the potato. Make sure your white rice flour is finely milled, otherwise you risk a gritty end product. Serve these with Vegan Bolognese (page 93) or panfried with some butter and sage leaves.

2 pounds (1 kg) Yukon Gold potatoes (or another floury to all-rounder variety)

Olive oil, for roasting

2⅓ cups (300 g) fine white rice flour

Scant ½ cup (50 g) tapioca flour, plus plenty extra to work the dough

1½ teaspoons fine salt

Olive oil

1. Preheat the oven to 350°F (180°C) and line a baking sheet with parchment paper. Lightly brush the potatoes with oil and space evenly on the baking sheet. Bake the potatoes for 40 minutes to 1 hour (depending on their size), until you can insert a knife through them. Remove from the oven and let cool.

2. While the potatoes are cooking, combine the flours and salt in a large mixing bowl.

3. Once the potatoes have cooled, use your hands to peel off the skins. (These can be sprayed with oil and baked, to make delicious potato skin chips.) Place the potatoes in a high-speed blender and blend until a sticky paste forms.

4. Transfer into the flour bowl. Using a spoon, and then your hands, combine into a shaggy, somewhat sticky but manageable ball of dough. If too sticky, add a little rice flour or tapioca flour.

5. Liberally flour a dry, clean bench space with tapioca flour and divide the dough into four balls. Use floured hands to roll each ball out into a long, thin rope, then cut the rope into gnocchi-size pieces with a sharp floured knife. Place on the baking sheet with space between each piece. Repeat with the remaining dough.

6. Bring a large pot of salted water to a boil, then carefully lower the gnocchi into the water, in batches of ten to twelve pieces at a time. Once they have risen to the surface, cook for 2 to 3 minutes before removing from the water. Test one piece and adjust the cooking time for the rest, if necessary.

7. Drain each piece of gnocchi well before transferring to a large mixing bowl, then drizzle lightly with olive oil so they don't stick to each other. Repeat until all the gnocchi is cooked, then serve.

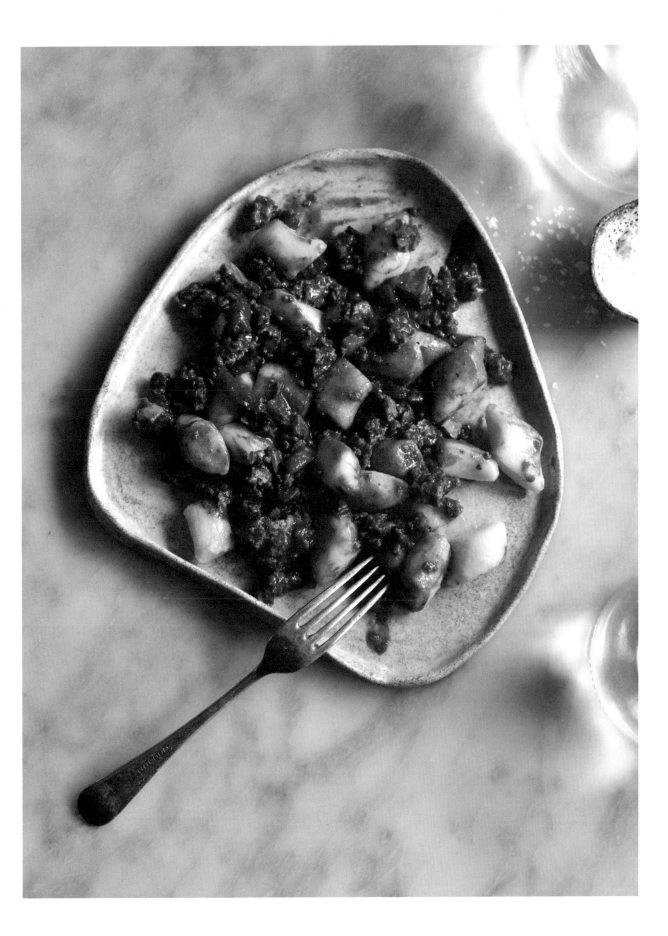

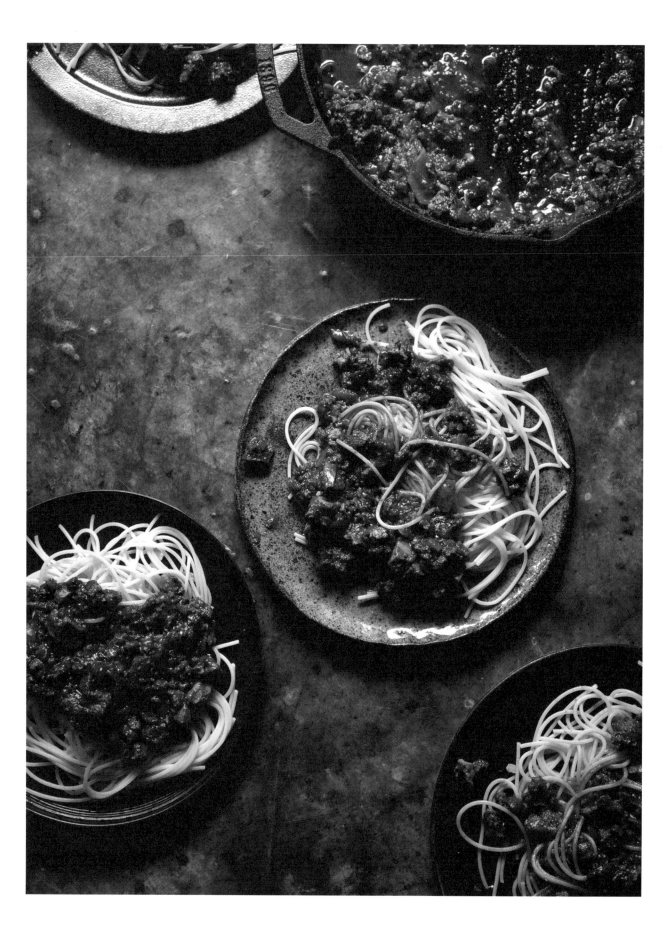

Vegan Bolognese

I know parents aren't supposed to play favorites, bu[...] Bolognese is undoubtedly my shining recipe child. By freezing and then defrosting tofu, it becomes alarmingly ground-meat-like in texture, resulting in a stunning con job of a Bolognese. Make sure your tofu is extra firm and that you don't tell your carnivore diners. Enjoy this on its own or over a bowl of gluten-free pasta. To keep it vegan, sprinkle nutritional yeast or vegan Parmesan on top. Personally, I like mine with some freshly grated vegetarian Parmesan.

2½ tablespoons olive oil

1 fennel bulb, finely chopped (for a lower-FODMAP option, use 2 medium carrots, finely chopped)

¼ cup (60 ml) FODMAP-Friendly Vegan Worcestershire Sauce (page 86; see Note)

2½ tablespoons balsamic vinegar

1 to 2 tablespoons gluten-free tamari

1 tablespoon gluten-free miso

2½ tablespoons tomato paste

½ cup (120 ml) red wine (you could probably substitute water, although the sauce won't be as rich)

Generous freshly cracked black pepper

One 28-ounce (794 g) can diced tomatoes

9 to 14 ounces (250 to 400 g) frozen, thawed, and drained tofu, depending how "meaty" you like your sauce, torn into small pieces

½ teaspoon ground allspice (optional)

1. Warm the olive oil in a large heavy-bottomed saucepan over medium heat. Add the fennel and cook for about 15 minutes, until it begins to shrivel and is starting to brown.

2. Add the Worcestershire sauce, vinegar, and tamari and stir to combine. Cook until the liquid has reduced.

3. Add the tomato paste and miso, and stir to combine. Add the wine and stir well, collecting all the little browned bits at the bottom.

4. Next, add the tomatoes and stir thoroughly. Season with pepper and add the tofu and allspice, if using. Cook for 10 to 15 minutes, until the tofu takes on some of the redness of the sauce and looks like ground meat. You can add a bit of water to thin the sauce out, if necessary.

5. Serve as desired.

Note: If you don't want to whip up a batch of the Worcestershire sauce just for this, simply use in its stead 2½ tablespoons apple cider vinegar, 2 tablespoons light brown sugar, and ½ teaspoon cinnamon, and increase the tamari to 2 or 2½ tablespoons. Some oregano and rosemary are particularly good additions for the Ultimate Vegetarian Lasagna (page 120).

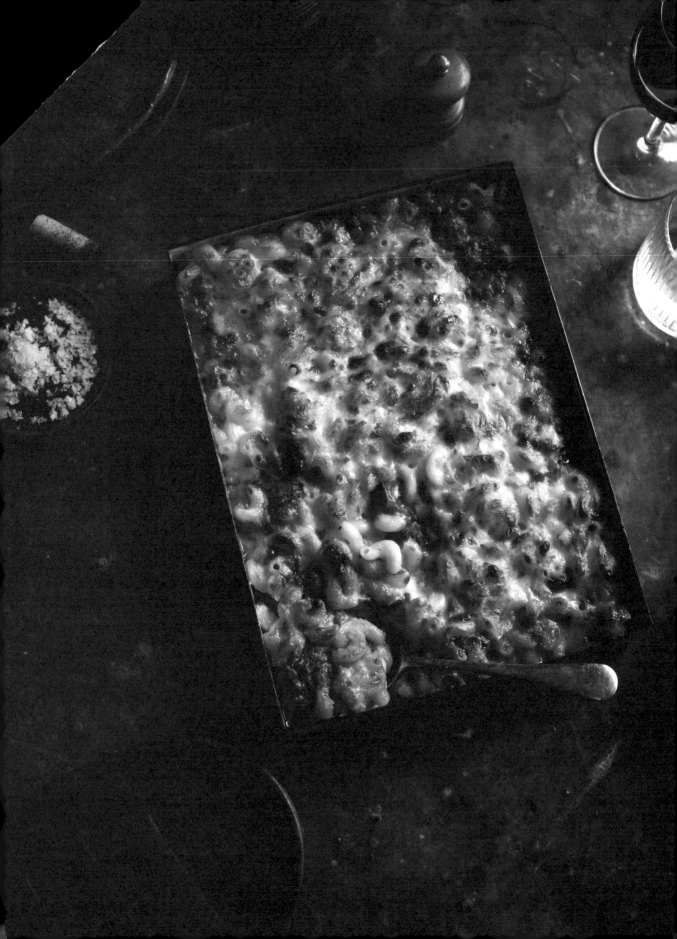

Vegetarian Bolognese Mac and Cheese Bake

MAKES 6 LARGE SERVINGS

Who is the genius who thought to combine mac and cheese with Bolognese-style sauce? While "hamburger helper" doesn't exist in Australia, I decided it was important for my personal growth to "do some research." My iteration uses my Vegan Bolognese combined with a low-lactose, gluten-free mac and cheese (which can stand alone as its own recipe).

5 tablespoons (75 g) butter

¼ cup (30 g) gluten-free cornstarch

3 cups (720 ml) cold milk of your choice

1 cup (100 g) freshly grated sharp aged cheddar, plus extra to top

½ cup (50 g) freshly grated Gruyère, plus extra to top

¾ cup (75 g) finely and freshly grated vegetarian Parmesan

Sea salt

Pinch of nutmeg (optional)

10 ounces (300 g) gluten-free macaroni, cooked al dente

1 recipe Vegan Bolognese (page 93)

1. Preheat the oven to 350°F (180°C).
2. Melt the butter in a large pot over medium-low heat, then whisk in the cornstarch. Allow the mixture to cook for a minute or so, then add the milk.
3. Whisk intermittently for about 10 minutes, until it is thick enough to coat the back of a spoon. Don't panic if it takes a while—it will get there with some patience.
4. Slowly incorporate the grated cheese. Season to taste and remove from the heat.
5. Add the cooked pasta to the cheese sauce and stir to combine.
6. Spread the Bolognese evenly in a 9 × 13 inch (23 × 33 cm) baking dish. Top this with the mac and cheese and finish with the extra cheese.
7. Bake in the oven for around 20 minutes, until the cheese is melted and bubbling. Turn the oven to broil and brown the top for 5 to 10 minutes, making sure you keep an eye on it.
8. Remove from the oven and serve.

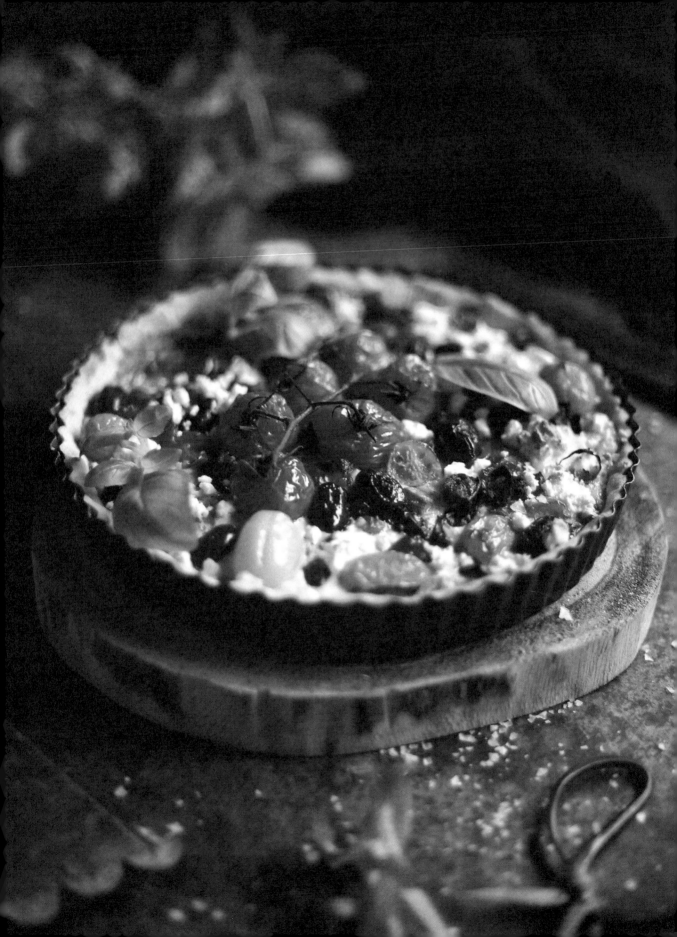

Roasted Vegetable Grain-Free Tart

SERVES 4 TO 6

This recipe pays homage to Ottolenghi's Very Full Tart. The man can make a good tart (and a good everything else, for that matter). Stuffed to the brim with Mediterranean-style roasted vegetables, low-FODMAP cheese, and olives, it takes a little time to prepare but sets you up for a few days of excellent dinners and lunches.

Filling

1 large (roughly 9 ounces/250 g) red bell pepper
Olive oil spray
2 cups (300 g) peeled, cubed kabocha squash, cut into ¾-inch (2 cm) pieces
2½ cups (200 g) cubed eggplant, cut into ¾-inch (2 cm) pieces
2½ tablespoons olive oil
2 teaspoons ground cinnamon
2 teaspoons ground nutmeg
½ teaspoon plus a pinch of sea salt
1 bunch basil, leaves only
⅔ cup (100 g) crumbled feta
1 fresh red chile, finely chopped
¼ cup (40 g) pitted kalamata olives
3 eggs
½ cup (125 ml) milk of your choice
Zest of ½ lemon
Cracked black pepper
⅔ cup (100 g) cherry tomatoes

Pastry crust

1 cup (120 g) tapioca flour
1½ cups (150 g) almond meal
½ cup (50 g) finely and freshly grated vegetarian Parmesan
7 tablespoons (100 g) butter
1 egg
Pinch of salt

1. Preheat the oven to 350°F (180°C). Grease and line a fluted 10-inch (26 cm) tart pan with a removable bottom.
2. **To make the filling,** place the bell pepper on a baking sheet, lightly spray with oil, and roast for 30 minutes or until the skin is blistering. Place in a bowl, cover with a kitchen towel, and set aside for a bit (the pepper will sweat and the skin will be a dream to remove). Remove and discard the skin and the seeds and slice the flesh into strips.
3. Combine the squash and eggplant in a bowl. Add the oil, cinnamon, nutmeg, and ½ teaspoon of the salt. Mix to ensure the vegetables are evenly coated in the oil and spices, and then divide evenly between two baking sheets. Roast for 20 to 30 minutes, until softened and nearly completely cooked through.
4. **To make the pastry crust,** place all the ingredients in a food processor and pulse until the mixture forms a ball of dough. Press the dough evenly into the prepared tart pan and use a fork to poke holes in the bottom of the pastry, to allow any air to escape. Bake in the oven for 10 minutes, or until lightly cooked.
5. **To assemble,** line the tart crust with half the basil leaves and about a third of the feta, followed by a second layer of basil (reserving some for garnish), then the chile, olives, and roasted vegetables.
6. Whisk together the eggs, milk, lemon zest, black pepper, and the remaining pinch of salt and pour evenly over the vegetables. Top with the tomatoes and remaining feta, then bake for 30 minutes, or until golden and the egg mixture has set. Garnish with the reserved basil and serve.

Vegan Laksa with Zucchini Noodles and Salt and Pepper Tofu

| SERVES 4 |

If there was ever a time to wear a bib to dinner, this is it. This delicious, comforting laksa is both FODMAP-friendly and vegan. It's also grain free courtesy of my using zucchini noodles, but if you're not quite as obnoxious as I am, feel free to use rice noodles.

Curry paste

5 red bird's eye chiles, seeded and finely chopped

2½ tablespoons (30 g) finely grated fresh galangal or ginger

6 to 10 small fresh curry leaves, finely chopped

1 tablespoon finely grated fresh turmeric

1 tablespoon finely grated lemongrass

2 teaspoons ground coriander

1 teaspoon gluten-free tamari

1 teaspoon fine salt

1 tablespoon vegetable oil

Laksa broth

4 cups (1 L) FODMAP-friendly vegetable stock (such as My Go-To Veggie Stock, page 62)

One 13.5-ounce (400 ml) can full-fat coconut milk

2 teaspoons light brown sugar

1 teaspoon tamarind paste (optional)

Salt and pepper tofu

Vegetable oil, for shallow frying

14 ounces (400 g) extra-firm tofu, well drained

2 teaspoons gluten-free cornstarch

1 teaspoon fine salt

1 teaspoon ground white pepper

To finish

1 bunch Chinese broccoli, roughly chopped

4 medium zucchini, made into noodles

Thai basil and Vietnamese mint

Chopped chiles, to taste

Lime wedges

1. **To make the curry paste,** blend together all the ingredients except the tamari, salt, and oil with a mortar and pestle or a food processor, until a smooth paste forms. Add the tamari and salt and continue to mix until smooth.

2. Place a large heavy-bottomed frying pan or wok over medium heat. Add the oil, then the curry paste. Lower the heat and cook for 5 minutes, or until fragrant. Add the sugar and continue cooking for a few minutes.

3. **To make the laksa broth,** add the stock to the curry paste and return to medium heat. Cook for 10 minutes, then add the coconut milk and continue to cook for an additional 10 minutes over low heat.

4. **To make the salt and pepper tofu,** while the laksa broth is cooking, chop the drained tofu into bite-size pieces. Combine the cornstarch, salt, and pepper in a large bowl and toss the tofu pieces in the mixture until they are well coated.

5. Heat a thin layer of oil in a nonstick saucepan over medium-high heat. In batches if necessary, cook the tofu on all sides until well browned. Transfer to a plate lined with paper towels or a cooling rack. Continue until you have cooked all the tofu.

6. **To finish,** a few minutes before serving, cook the Chinese broccoli: If using this or a bok choy–type vegetable, you can steam it in a separate pot beforehand, or just cook in the laksa broth and wait a few extra minutes.

7. Add the zucchini noodles and cook for a minute or so, until they are just softening.

8. Divide the mixture between four large bowls and top each with the tofu, herbs, and chiles. Serve immediately with lime wedges.

Note: You can freeze the laksa if you'd like, but I'd recommend freezing either the paste or the soup, without the zucchini noodles and tofu. Those are best fresh.

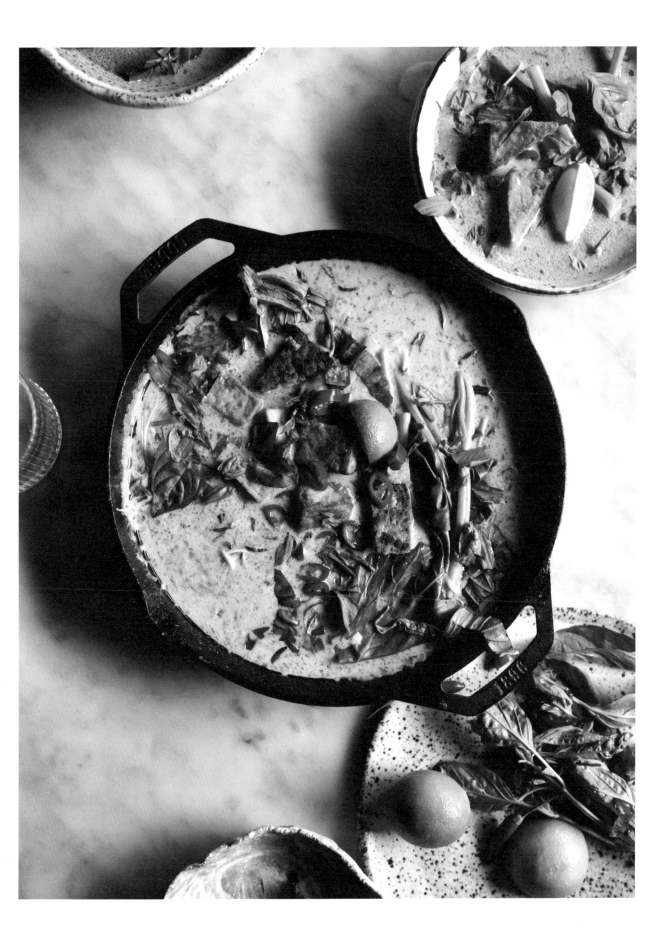

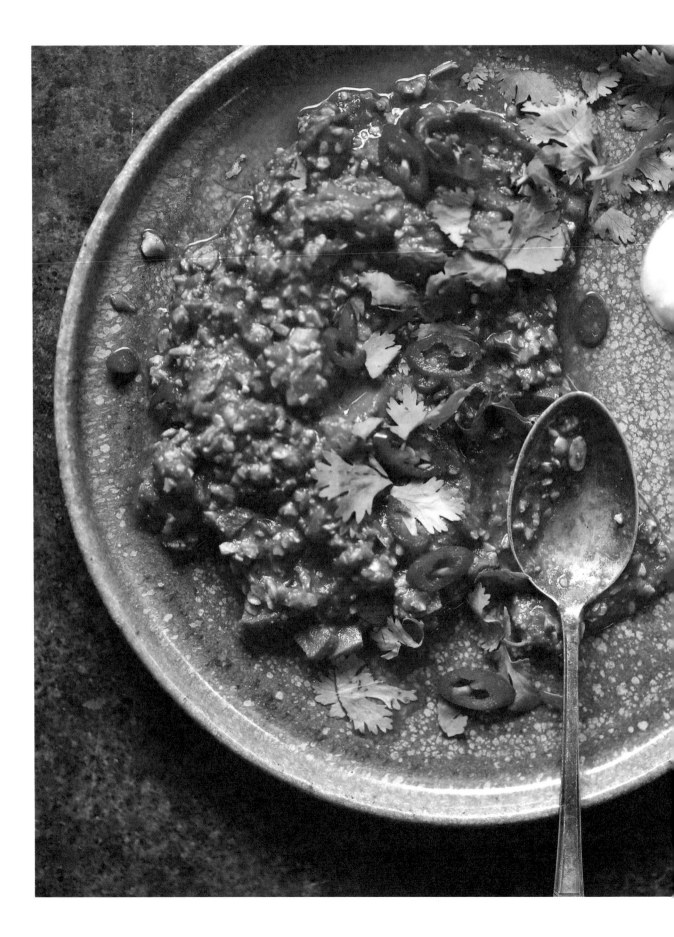

Tempeh Chili

SERVES 2

Forgive me if I'm using more tempeh than you'd like, but it really is such a great low-**FODMAP** alternative to beans, even though it's still officially a bean itself. It's a **FODMAP** miracle! This chili can be served in the same way as you would a beef chili: in tacos, with rice, or straight up in a bowl. The coconut yogurt is an exotic alternative to sour cream, but you can use sour cream if dairy isn't a grievous issue for you.

3 Asian eggplants (1¼ pounds/ 600 g)

2 red bell peppers (7 ounces/ 400 g)

1 fresh red chile

2½ tablespoons vegetable oil (olive oil is OK, if that's all you have)

1 tablespoon ground cumin

1 tablespoon smoked paprika

2 teaspoons ground cinnamon

1 teaspoon ground coriander

½ teaspoon red pepper flakes, or to taste

One 14.5 ounce (411 g) can diced tomatoes (no salt or added flavors)

2 teaspoons light brown sugar

8 ounces (225 g) tempeh, chopped or very roughly pulsed in a food processor

1 bunch cilantro (stems chopped; reserve leaves for serving)

1 carrot, chopped

1 zucchini, chopped

1 cup (250 ml) FODMAP-friendly vegetable stock (such as My Go-To Veggie Stock, page 62)

To serve (all optional)
Lime wedges
Coconut yogurt or sour cream
Fresh red chile, finely sliced

1. Over an open flame (ideally a gas stove or a grill, but a broiler will suffice if you don't have either of these), char your eggplants, bell peppers, and chile. Use tongs to turn them and continue charring until they are completely black, blistering, and peeling all over. Transfer to a bowl and cover with water. Once they have cooled slightly, peel and discard the charred skin, and chop the flesh roughly.

2. Heat the oil in a large saucepan over medium heat and add the spices. Stir for a couple of minutes until fragrant, then add the tomatoes, sugar, tempeh, cilantro stems, carrot, zucchini, and the charred vegetables.

3. Stir thoroughly to combine and allow the chili to cook for a few minutes, until bubbling and fragrant. Stir in the stock, then cover and cook over medium heat for 20 to 30 minutes, stirring intermittently.

4. Serve with a squeeze of lime and some coconut yogurt, if desired, and sprinkle with some fresh chile and the cilantro leaves, if you like (it is the most controversial herb, after all).

Zucchini, Ricotta, and Herb Tart

**MAKES ONE
10-INCH (26 CM)
TART**

This tart reminds me of the snake Kaa's hypnotic eyes in the *Jungle Book*, which is possibly why I love it so much. It is a little time consuming (we can call it kitchen meditation) but a real showstopper once complete. The zucchini may leak liquid—you can either drain the slices well ahead of time (sprinkling with fine salt to extract moisture before patting dry), or you can use a paper towel to suck the moisture off the top of the tart after it cooks. That's the infinitely easier option.

Tart crust

1½ cups (150 g) almond meal
1 scant cup (100 g) tapioca flour
5½ tablespoons (80 g) butter
1 egg
1 to 2 teaspoons olive oil
¼ cup (25 g) freshly grated
   vegetarian Parmesan

Filling

2 cups (500 g) ricotta (see
   Lactose-Free "Ricotta" Toasts,
   page 46)
1 cup (100 g) freshly grated
   vegetarian Parmesan
½ cup (75 g) crumbled feta
2 teaspoons ground nutmeg
Sea salt, to taste
Cracked black pepper, to taste
Red pepper flakes, to taste
2 eggs
1 bunch dill, finely chopped
1 bunch mint, finely chopped
¼ to ⅓ cup (35 to 50 g) capers
3 to 4 medium zucchini

1. Preheat the oven to 350°F (180°C). Grease a 10-inch (26 cm) tart pan.
2. **To make the crust,** combine all the ingredients in a food processor and pulse, until it comes together into a dough. Press the dough into the prepared pan until it is nice and snug. Poke a few fork holes in the base to allow air to escape, then pop it in the oven for 10 to 15 minutes, until golden. Remove from the oven and let cool.
3. **Meanwhile, to make the filling,** loosen the ricotta with ½ cup (120 ml) water, stir in the Parmesan, feta, nutmeg, salt, black pepper, and red pepper flakes, then mix in the eggs. Fold in the herbs and capers.
4. Use a mandoline to finely slice your zucchini lengthwise. Then, use a knife to slice each of those thin slices in half lengthwise (so you have two long slices instead of one).
5. **To finish,** pour the cheesy ricotta mixture into the pastry and smooth it over.
6. Now for the fun part. Take one zucchini ribbon and curl it around itself, until it becomes a tight circle. Plonk it down in the middle of the tart, pressing it down into the ricotta a little. Continue to wrap your zucchini around this center circle, until you have completely covered the tart in zucchini.
7. Bake in the oven for 40 minutes to 1 hour, until set and lightly browned.
8. Gently slice and serve!

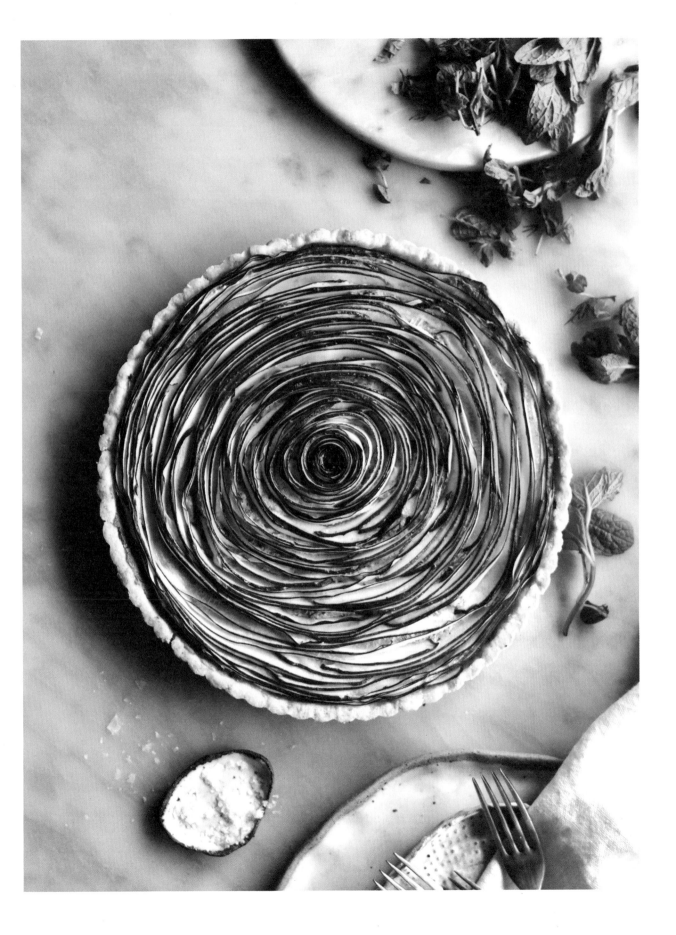

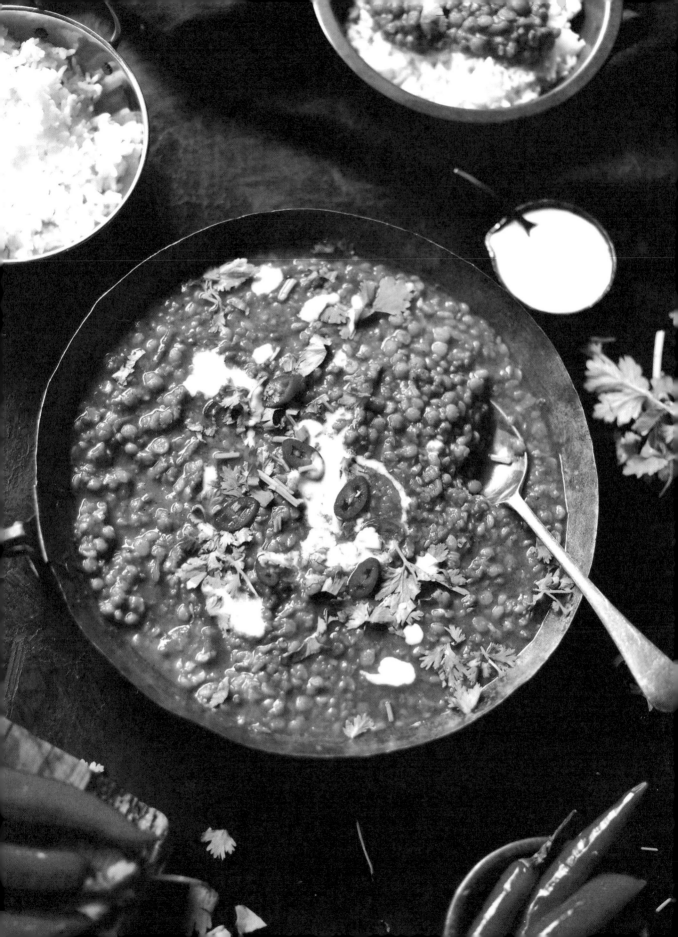

Chana Dal

SERVES 6 TO 8

Legumes? Am I serious? Yes, I am very serious. And very seriously into this dal. By leaching the oligo fructans out of the chana dal (otherwise known as split chickpeas or Bengal gram), it becomes FODMAP-friendly in half-cup servings. Because of the somewhat tedious nature of the process, I've created this recipe to yield a large serving—perfect for the freezer, perfect for this trendy thing called "meal prep." Seriously, thank me later.

2 cups (400 g) chana dal (split chickpeas)
2 bay leaves
1 cinnamon stick
½ teaspoon chili powder
2½ teaspoons garam masala
1½ teaspoons ground turmeric
2½ tablespoons (40 g) butter or ghee
1½ cups (300 g) chopped tomatoes
2-inch (6 cm) piece fresh ginger, finely chopped or grated
1 teaspoon ground cumin
1 teaspoon ground cinnamon
1 teaspoon coriander seeds
½ teaspoon fennel seeds
½ teaspoon red pepper flakes, or to taste
4 cardamom pods, seeds removed and husks discarded
2 teaspoons sea salt
Cracked black pepper
1½ cups (375 ml) boiling water

To serve
Rice
Cilantro leaves (optional)
Coconut yogurt (optional)
Fresh red chile, finely sliced (optional)

1. Cover the split chickpeas with water in a large bowl and set aside for at least 1 hour. Drain, rinse well, and transfer to a large saucepan with fresh water. Bring to a boil and keep on high heat for 10 minutes. Drain and rinse again, then add fresh water and the bay leaves, cinnamon stick, chili powder, and ½ teaspoon each of the garam masala and turmeric. Cook over medium heat for at least 30 minutes, until the liquid has mostly absorbed and the split chickpeas are soft. Remove from the heat and drain.

2. Heat a large saucepan over medium heat and melt the butter. Add the tomatoes and ginger and cook until soft, 5 to 10 minutes, adding a splash of water if necessary.

3. Add the remaining 2 teaspoons garam masala and 1 teaspoon turmeric, the cumin, ground cinnamon, coriander, fennel, red pepper flakes, and cardamom. Season with the salt and some pepper and cook for a minute or two until fragrant. Add the split chickpeas and the boiling water, then stir well and cook over low heat for 15 to 20 minutes, until the liquid has thickened slightly and the dish is bubbling and fragrant. Remove the bay leaves and cinnamon stick.

4. Serve ½ cup portions with rice and top with cilantro leaves, a spoonful of coconut yogurt, and fresh red chile, if desired.

Involtini

Involtini will forever be associated with celebrations for me. My mum has always made them as the vegetarian contribution for family get-togethers. I also celebrate the mere fact that I have them in the fridge because once they're made, you've got dinner and lunch sorted for a week.

2 pounds (1 kg) ripe tomatoes, chopped (about 5 ½ cups), or one 28-ounce (794 g) can diced tomatoes with no added salt or flavors

3 to 4 eggplants (about 2 pounds/ 1 kg)

Pinch of sea salt, plus extra for the eggplant

2 cups (500 g) fresh ricotta (see Lactose-Free "Ricotta" Toasts, page 46)

1 bunch dill, finely chopped

1 bunch mint, finely chopped

½ bunch basil, finely chopped

1 cup (100 g) grated vegetarian Parmesan

¼ cup (35 g) capers, drained

2½ tablespoons olive oil

2 teaspoons ground nutmeg

1 teaspoon red pepper flakes

Pinch of cracked black pepper

Cheddar cheese, to finish

1. Heat a large frying pan over a medium heat and add the tomatoes and 1 cup (250 ml) water. Cook until the tomatoes break down and have a pasta-sauce consistency.

2. Meanwhile, slice the eggplants lengthwise about ½ inch (1 cm) thick—thin enough to roll, but thick enough to hold the ricotta. Place the slices in a colander over the sink and salt generously. This will help to remove excess moisture.

3. Combine the ricotta, herbs, Parmesan, capers, oil, spices, and the remaining pinch of salt in a large bowl. Adjust the seasoning if necessary, and then set aside.

4. Spread the cooked tomatoes over the bottom of a large casserole dish. Take a slice of eggplant and spoon a rough tablespoon of the ricotta mixture onto one end of the eggplant slice. Roll up the eggplant and then place into the tomatoes, seam side down. Repeat with the remaining eggplant and ricotta.

5. Once the involtini are all assembled and packed into the dish, grate a generous amount of cheddar on top. Bake for around 30 minutes, until bubbling and brown. Remove from the oven, let cool slightly, and serve.

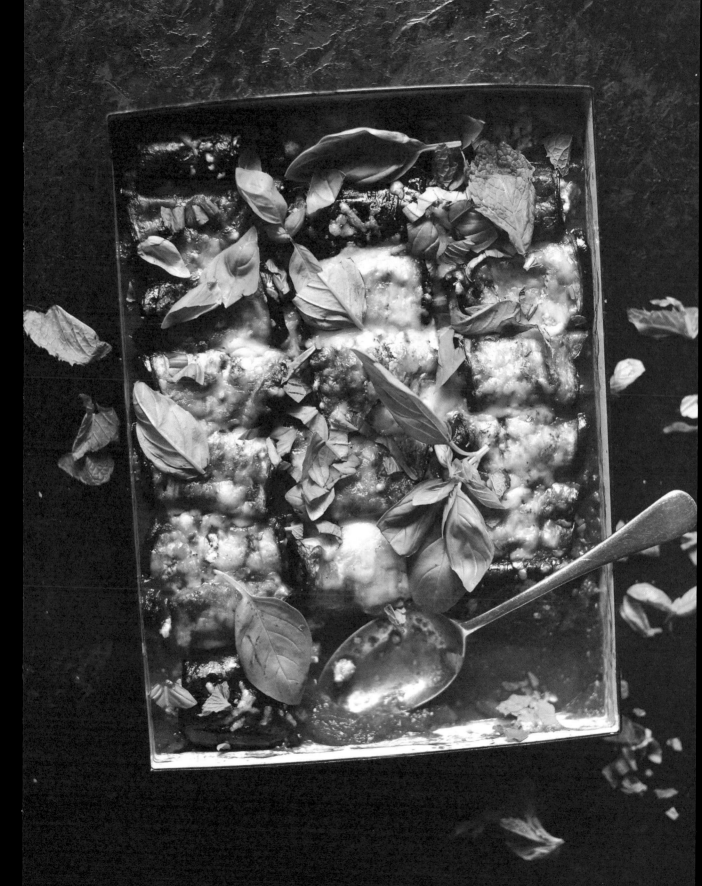

Pepper, Pesto, and Goat Cheese Galette

SERVES
4 TO 6

If you followed me on Instagram for, I don't know, a week, you'd see that I'm a huge fan of making tarts. What I despise, however, is the physical act of pressing the pastry into the tart pan—I have no patience, and no appreciation of fine details. The solution? A galette! Essentially a free-form tart, the trusty galette eliminates the worst part of tart making, and looks beautiful and rustic while doing so. Because the only thing I like more than putting minimal effort in is looking like I've put a lot of effort in.

Pastry

1 cup (100 g) hazelnut meal or almond meal
1 cup (130 g) fine brown rice flour
½ cup (60 g) tapioca flour
5 tablespoons (75 g) butter, diced
½ cup (50 g) freshly grated vegetarian Parmesan
2 eggs, plus 1 extra egg yolk (see Note)
½ teaspoon sea salt

Pepper filling

4 bell peppers (about 1½ pounds/ 750 g)
2½ to 4 tablespoons FODMAP-Friendly Pesto (page 121)
⅓ cup (50 g) crumbled goat cheese or feta
Olive oil spray

1. **To make the pastry,** combine all the ingredients in a food processor and pulse until a dough forms. Shape this into a ball, wrap in beeswax or plastic wrap, and refrigerate for at least an hour, until it feels nice and firm.
2. **To start the filling,** preheat the oven to 350°F (180°C). Line a baking sheet with parchment paper.
3. Cut the peppers in half, remove the seeds, and assemble them on the baking sheet. Roast in the oven for 30 minutes, or until the flesh has softened and the skin is blistered. Transfer to a bowl and cover with a kitchen towel. Once cooled, remove the skins, tear the peppers into fat strips, and set aside.
4. **To assemble the galette,** place the dough between two large sheets of parchment paper and gently roll out into an oval shape (about 12 × 10 inches/30 × 25 cm). Peel the top layer of paper off and then gently slide the pastry, atop the remaining piece of parchment paper, onto a large baking sheet.
5. Spread the pesto over the pastry and sprinkle half the cheese in a central oval shape. Lay the peppers over the cheese, leaving enough room to pull the pastry edges up over the outer edges of the pepper layer.
6. Use the sheet of parchment paper to gently pull the pastry up around the pepper, one edge at a time. Press down firmly to secure the pastry to the pepper slices, and work your way around, pulling all the pastry edges up to form a galette.
7. Sprinkle with the remaining cheese and spray lightly with oil. Transfer the galette to the oven and cook for 30 to 35 minutes, until the pastry is golden and the filling is bubbly. Give the peppers an extra spray of oil if it looks too brown at any point. Remove from the oven, slice lengthwise, and serve.

Note: A traditional galette does not contain any eggs, but this version does, as the dry ingredients used here tend to be quite thirsty.

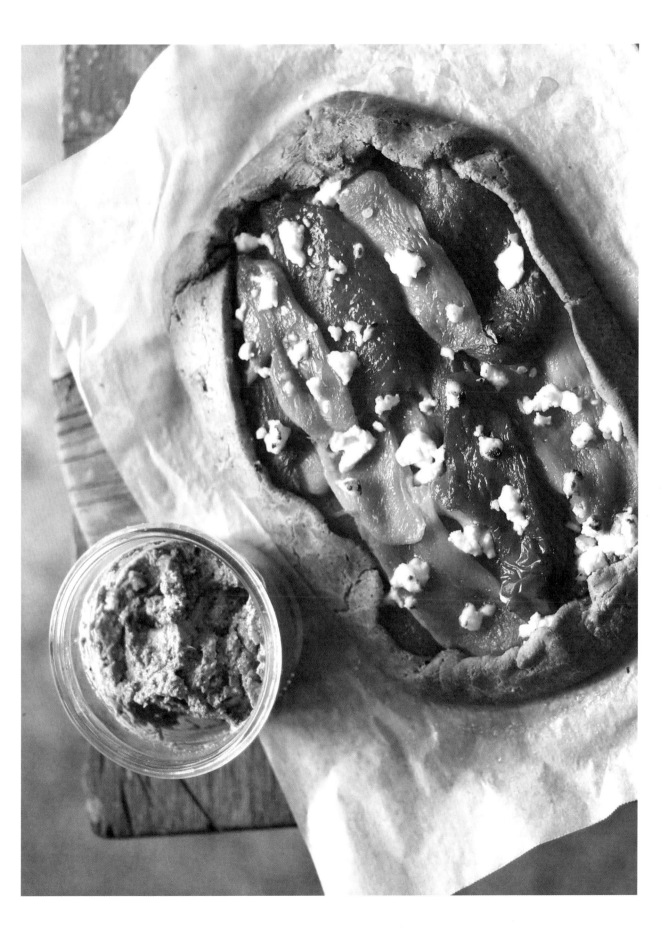

Shahi Paneer

SERVES 4

I have been a fervent devotee of shahi paneer since I was a little university student, whose only dietary considerations were if said dish was an appropriate hangover cure. (Spoiler alert: This was, and still is.) To honor my past, I've created a shahi paneer that is decidedly more FODMAP-friendly: It uses fennel (or carrots) as an aromatic base, nixing the need for onion or garlic. If you'd like to make a vegan version, simply substitute the paneer with cubed tofu and the cream and milk with plant-based alternatives. Serve as is, or with rice or Coconut Flatbreads (page 111).

14 ounces (400 g) paneer, diced into bite-size pieces

⅓ cup (80 ml) peanut oil, plus extra as needed

1 large or 2 small fennel bulbs, or 2 large carrots, finely diced

1 smallish green chile, finely chopped

2-inch (6 cm) piece fresh ginger, finely chopped

14 cardamom pods, crushed and husks discarded

1 tablespoon plus 1 teaspoon ground coriander

2 teaspoons garam masala whole spices (see Note)

2 teaspoons ground turmeric

2 pinches of ground cinnamon

2 good pinches of cayenne

2 good pinches of fine salt

2 good pinches of cracked black pepper

2 teaspoons coconut sugar or light brown sugar

4 tomatoes, diced

1 cup (250 ml) lactose-free milk

½ cup (125 g) lactose-free cream or heavy cream

Fresh red chile, finely sliced (optional)

Lime wedges (optional)

1. In a medium saucepan over medium-high heat, dry-fry the paneer cubes for 8 to 10 minutes, until they have a nice brown color and sealed edges. Set aside.

2. Rinse the saucepan, if necessary, before returning it to low heat with the oil and fennel. Cook the fennel for 15 minutes. Add a splash of water if the fennel starts to stick at any point.

3. In the meantime, combine the chile and ginger in a large mortar and pound with the pestle into a paste. Add all of the spices, the sugar, and 2 teaspoons water, and pound again. Eventually it will come together into a curry paste.

4. The fennel should be done by now, so transfer it to a bowl and put the saucepan back on the heat. Put the tomatoes in the saucepan and cook over medium heat until they lose their form and take on a pasta-sauce consistency. Spoon the curry paste into the pan and stir into the tomatoes. Add a little bit of oil to ensure it doesn't burn.

5. Return the fennel to the pan and cook for a few more minutes until everything is combined and fragrant.

6. Pour the mixture into a food processor, allow it to cool a bit (blending hot ingredients is generally not a fun time), and blitz into a lovely, smooth sauce, 2 to 3 minutes.

7. Back into the pan we go, this time stirring in the milk and 1 cup (250 ml) water. Bring to a simmer, then add the paneer cubes, mixing well to combine. Cook for a few minutes, then stir in the cream. Remove from the heat and serve with the red chile and lime wedges, for squeezing, if desired.

Note: Whole garam masala can be found at most Indian or Asian grocers. It's the whole-spice form of the ground garam masala you buy at the supermarket. Using freshly ground spices gives dishes a more intense flavor, but if the only thing standing between you and shahi paneer is finding whole garam masala, then stick with the ground version.

Coconut Flatbreads

MAKES 6 TO 8
FLATBREADS

Things that get old really quickly: watching people eat roti while you cannot. This isn't quite roti, but it's not quite having no roti either. You can serve these with a curry or just inhale them on their own.

½ cup (60 g) fine white rice flour

¼ cup (25 g) almond meal

¼ cup (40 g) potato starch

1¼ cups (310 ml) coconut milk (make sure it doesn't contain added inulin)

1 teaspoon ground garam masala

1 teaspoon fine salt

1 egg

1 teaspoon butter, for frying

1. Whisk all the ingredients, except the butter, together in a medium bowl.
2. Heat a nonstick frying pan over medium-high heat, until hot. Melt the butter and pour in about ¼ cup (60 ml) of the batter for each flatbread.
3. Fry for a minute or so, until the surface is covered in bubbles, and then gently flip over and cook the other side. Transfer to a plate and cover to keep warm until serving. Repeat with the rest of the batter.

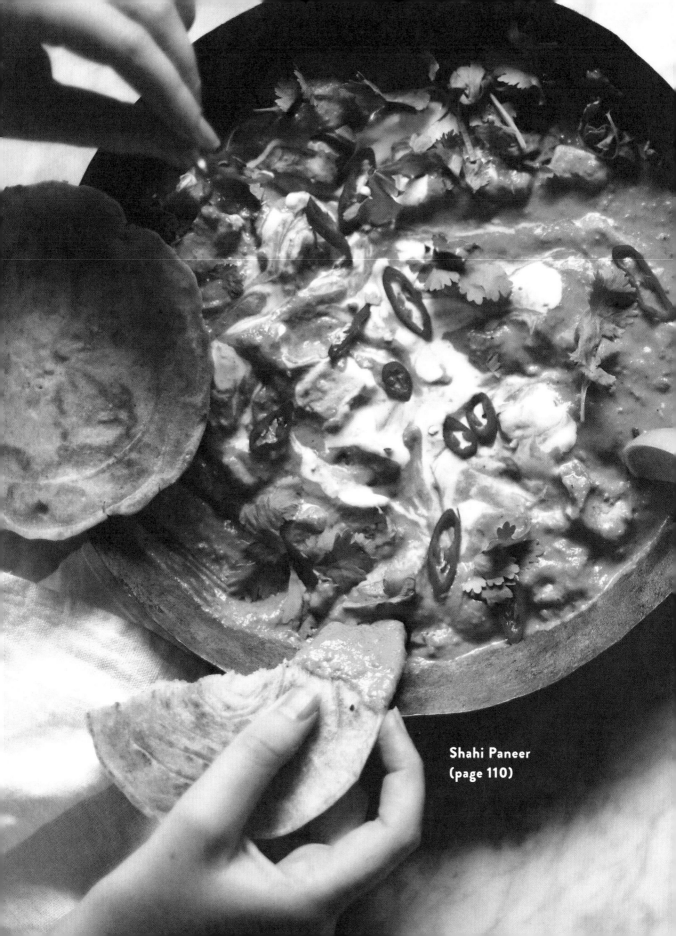

Shahi Paneer
(page 110)

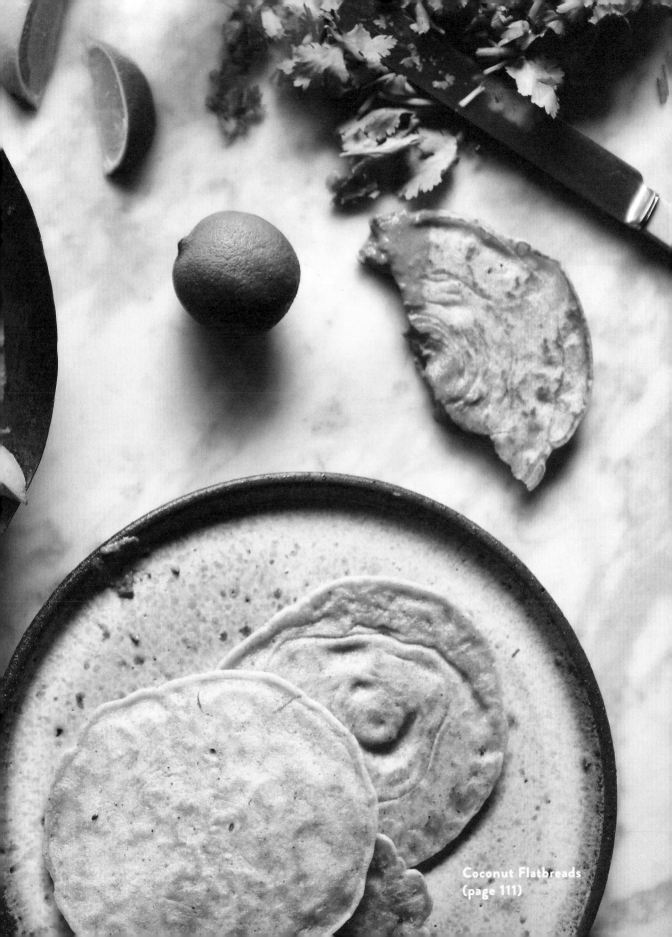

Coconut Flatbreads
(page 111)

Tofu (Run) Amok

I can basically guarantee that if you've been to Cambodia, you've fallen in love with amok—a fragrant coconut-based curry perfumed with makrut and turmeric. Amok is hard to describe, but even harder to forget (Hallmark, are you hiring?). This a vegan version of the Cambodian delicacy, one that uses tofu instead of fish. I like to use a microplane for the grated ingredients in this recipe, but if you're chopping them, do so incredibly finely. Serve as is, or with rice.

Curry paste

2½ teaspoons finely grated fresh galangal

1 teaspoon finely grated fresh turmeric

6 makrut lime leaves, finely chopped

½ teaspoon finely grated makrut lime zest (see page 82)

2 lemongrass stems, white parts only, finely grated

2 teaspoons coconut sugar

½ teaspoon hot sauce

½ teaspoon fine salt, plus extra as needed

Tofu amok

2½ tablespoons peanut oil

1 cup (250 ml) coconut milk (make sure it doesn't contain inulin)

1 to 2 teaspoons gluten-free tamari

10 ounces (300 g) tofu, cut into large chunks

To serve (all optional)

Cilantro leaves

Fresh red chile, finely sliced

Coconut cream

1. **To make the curry paste,** combine the galangal, turmeric, makrut lime leaves and zest, and lemongrass in a mortar or food processor and grind to a paste. Keep in mind that this is a small volume of paste, so your food processor might struggle.

2. Add the sugar, hot sauce, salt, and 2 teaspoons water, and continue to grind until everything is well incorporated.

3. **To make the tofu amok,** heat the oil in a large saucepan over medium heat. Add the curry paste and cook until fragrant. Add the coconut milk and tamari and stir until the paste is combined and the coconut milk is a vibrant yellow.

4. Add the tofu to the curry and cook for around 10 minutes, until the tofu is heated through. Turn off the heat and leave to cool for a few minutes.

5. Serve with some cilantro leaves, chile, and a little coconut cream, if you like.

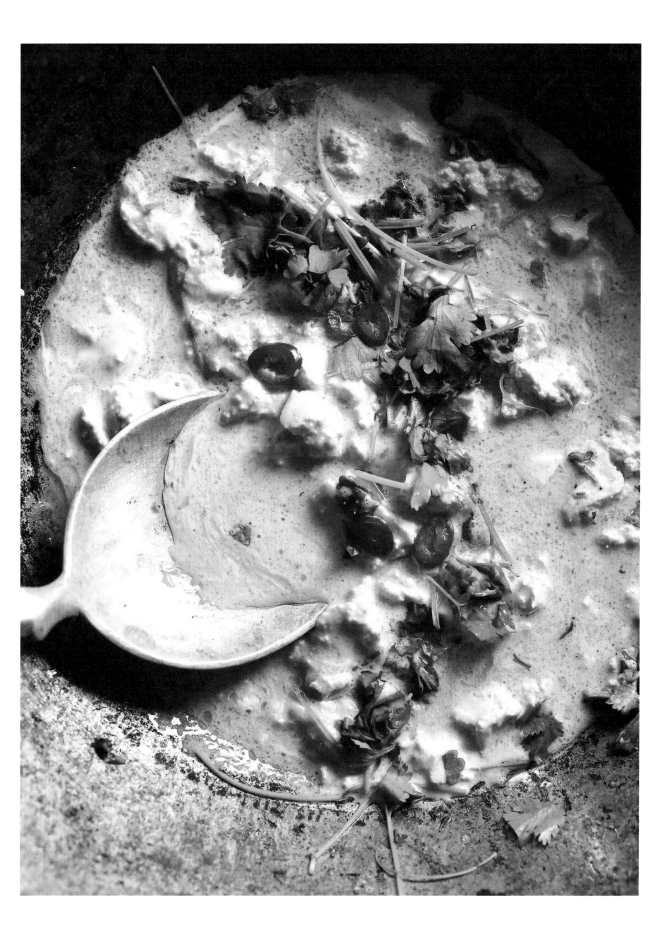

Vegetarian Enchiladas

SERVES 6 TO 8

There are two main food groups whose lack of variety in Australia gives me much grief: potatoes and chiles. So, straight out of the gate: This is a cheater's version of "enchilada-style" sauce. I don't have access to half as many chile varieties here, so cheater's it had to be. If you'd like to make a more authentic version, do so without any onion or garlic.

Vegan taco filling

1 pound (450 g) firm tofu, frozen, thawed, and drained
¼ cup (60 ml) olive oil
1 medium fennel bulb, finely chopped
2½ tablespoons light brown sugar
1 tablespoon smoked paprika
2 to 3 teaspoons ground cumin
2 teaspoons dried oregano
1 teaspoon ground cinnamon
¼ to ½ teaspoon red pepper flakes
1 to 2 tablespoons cocoa powder (optional)
¼ cup (60 ml) apple cider vinegar
¼ cup (65 g) tomato paste
2½ tablespoons gluten-free tamari
One 28-ounce (794 g) can whole peeled tomatoes
Generous freshly cracked black pepper

Enchilada sauce

1 tablespoon ground cumin
1 tablespoon dried oregano
1 tablespoon smoked paprika
1 to 3 teaspoons ground chile
1 teaspoon ground cinnamon
1 teaspoon cocoa powder (optional)
1 teaspoon sea salt flakes
¼ cup (60 ml) olive oil
2½ tablespoons gluten-free cornstarch
¼ cup (65 g) tomato paste
1 tablespoon apple cider vinegar
½ teaspoon gluten-free tamari, to taste (only if you need a salty umami kick)

1. **To make the vegan taco filling,** break the tofu into little pieces, similar to the size and texture of cooked ground meat. Set aside.
2. Heat the oil in a large frying pan over medium-low heat until shimmering and add the fennel. Cook for 10 to 15 minutes, until the fennel is bronzed and looks like caramelized onion.
3. Add the sugar, spices, and cocoa, if using, and stir thoroughly to coat. Next, add the vinegar, tomato paste, and tamari. The mixture will sizzle and evaporate rapidly as the liquid hits the pan, so work quickly. Add the canned tomatoes and stir thoroughly to combine. Season with black pepper and other spices, if needed.
4. Add the tofu and stir thoroughly to coat. Cook for 5 minutes or until the tofu has completely taken on the color of the sauce. Transfer to a bowl and set aside.
5. **To make the enchilada sauce,** combine the spices, cocoa, and salt in a small bowl.
6. Heat the oil over medium-low heat in the same pan you used for the tofu. Once the oil is shimmering, stir in the cornstarch until it forms a paste, about a minute or so.
7. Stir in the spices. Mix in the tomato paste, vinegar, and tamari, then pour in the stock. Stir to combine and cook for 5 to 10 minutes, until it has thickened. Remove from the heat.
8. **To finish,** ladle about half the enchilada sauce into a large rectangular baking dish. Preheat the oven to 350°F (180°C).
9. Heat a thin layer of oil in a nonstick pan over medium-high heat until shimmery. I like to do this next part in an assembly-line format, working with one tortilla at a time: Cook each side quickly until it is bubbly and coated in oil. Stuff the tortilla generously with tofu, placing the tofu toward one side of the tortilla, not in the center. Roll the tortilla and place it seam side down into the dish. Repeat with the remaining tortillas until the dish is full.

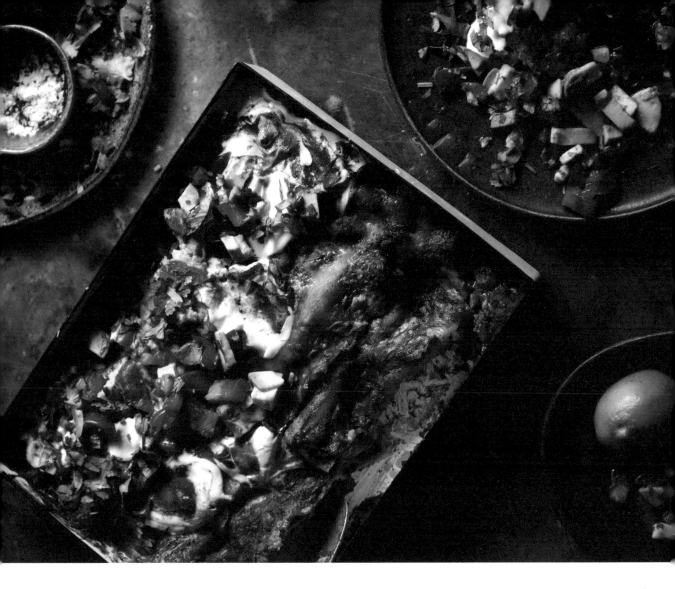

3 cups (700 ml) FODMAP-friendly
vegetable stock (such as My Go-To
Veggie Stock, page 62)
Generous freshly cracked black pepper

To finish
Neutral oil, for frying
16 white corn tortillas
Freshly grated cheddar cheese
(smoked would be delicious)
1 to 2 large tomatoes, chopped
1 to 2 ripe avocados, chopped
Cilantro, chopped
Lime wedges
Sea salt flakes
Sour cream (lactose-free or vegan, if
you'd prefer)

10. Top the tortillas with the remaining enchilada sauce
and then cover with freshly grated cheese. Bake in the
oven for 15 to 20 minutes, until the cheese melts and
browns.
11. While you're waiting, make a salsa by combining the
tomato, avocado, and cilantro in a large bowl. Spritz
with lime juice and season with salt.
12. To serve, either plonk the salsa on top or serve it as a
side. Scatter with a generous amount of sour cream, if
you like, and go to town.

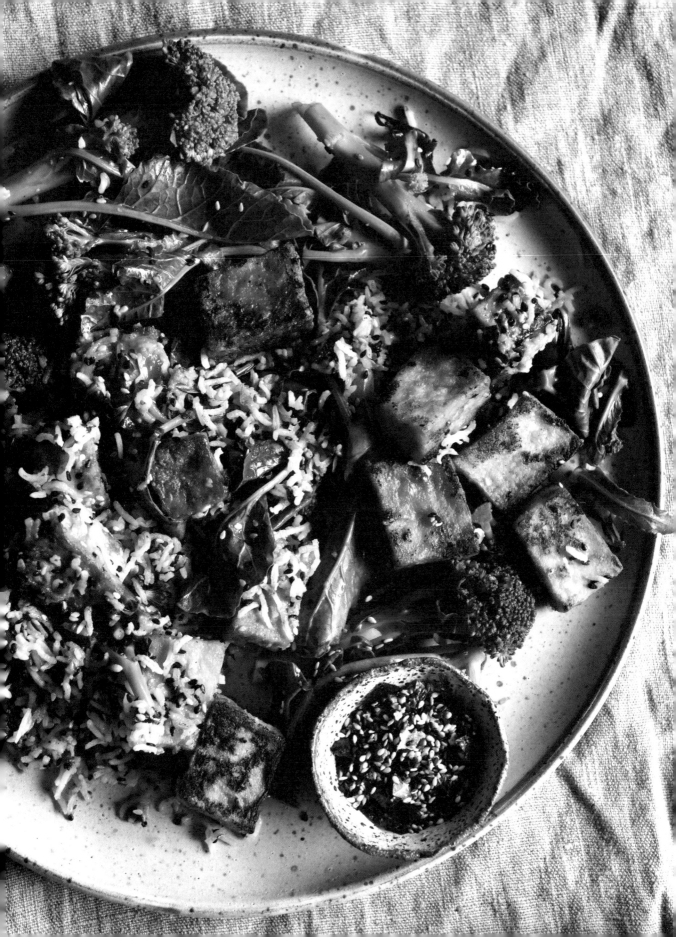

Vegan Furikake Rice Bowls with Crispy Miso Tofu and Broccolini

SERVES 2 TO 4, depending on how hungry you are

I bet you five dollars I can get you hooked on furikake, if you're not already. Although the name sounds a little like something I learned about through Cards Against Humanity, it's actually a sweet and salty sesame and seaweed condiment. The traditional recipe uses various iterations of seafood and/or some harder-to-come-by ingredients—this is a simplified vegan version. Please note: I will not honor this bet (although I don't think I'll need to).

Furikake rice bowls

½ cup (65 g) white sesame seeds
½ cup (65 g) black sesame seeds
1 to 2 sheets nori, chopped into tiny bits
2 to 3 teaspoons coconut sugar or light brown sugar
1 teaspoon sea salt flakes
1 cup (roughly 200 g) white rice
14 ounces (400 g) broccolini (about 2 bunches)

Crispy miso tofu

2½ tablespoons gluten-free cornstarch
Vegetable oil, for frying
16 ounces (450 g) firm tofu, pressed (see Note) and cubed
2 tablespoons gluten-free miso
1 tablespoon grated fresh ginger
1 tablespoon maple syrup
1 tablespoon toasted sesame oil
1 tablespoon gluten-free tamari
Refined sesame oil, for cooking (optional)

1. **To make the furikake rice bowls,** toast the sesame seeds in a saucepan over medium heat, until they are golden in color. Add the nori and toast for a minute or so. Finally, add the sugar and salt and stir until the mixture becomes a little bit sticky. Remove from the heat and set aside.

2. Cook the rice using your preferred method, then set aside.

3. While the rice cooks, boil a pot of water and blanch the broccolini until just cooked, then drain immediately.

4. **To make the tofu,** coat it in the cornstarch and heat the vegetable oil in a frying pan over medium-high heat. Fry in batches, intermittently turning until all sides are brown. Set aside on a cooling rack.

5. Whisk all the remaining ingredients together in a large bowl. Set aside.

6. You have a few options: You can combine the rice and broccolini (some chopped, some whole, for texture) in a large bowl, and toss in furikake to taste (keeping in mind that the sesame seeds may extend the FODMAP limits). Toss the tofu in the miso sauce and then serve either mixed together or separately. Alternatively, you can heat a saucepan over medium heat with a splash of refined sesame oil and add the broccolini, giving it a bit of char and crunch. From there, you can char the edges of the miso-covered tofu, for extra crispiness, and you could even toss the rice in, for a few crispy grains. The world is your delightfully sesame-seaweed-flavored oyster. Let's not talk about how many times I've used this line.

Note: Press the tofu by placing it between sheets of paper towel with a heavy object on top. Drain the tofu for an hour or so, and change the paper towel at least once in the process.

Ultimate Vegetarian Lasagna

SERVES 6 TO 8

Heaven is a place on Earth: It's wherever someone has made lasagna and frozen portions for lazy dinners. This number is a little time consuming, but it takes all the best elements of a baked dish and combines them into one comforting, filling, and delicious lasagna. There's a vegan version on my website, if that's more your speed.

Roasted vegetables

4 red bell peppers (or a jar of roasted bell peppers, with no added onion or garlic)

3½ cups (500 g) peeled, cubed kabocha squash

1 or 2 zucchini, cubed

Olive oil

Fine salt

Cracked black pepper

Béchamel

7 tablespoons (100 g) butter

⅓ cup (40 g) gluten-free cornstarch

4 cups (1 L) lactose-free whole milk

1 cup (100 g) freshly and finely grated vegetarian Parmesan

1 cup (100 g) grated smoked mozzarella, plus extra for topping

Fine salt

Good pinch of nutmeg (optional, but delicious)

To finish

One 10-ounce (283 g) package gluten-free oven-ready lasagna noodles

1 recipe Vegan Bolognese (page 93)

1 to 2 large handfuls spinach (see Note)

1 bunch basil (see Note)

Fine salt

Cracked black pepper

1. **To make the roasted vegetables,** preheat the oven to 350°F (180°C). Line two baking sheets with parchment paper, arrange the peppers on one, and place on the top rack of the oven. Arrange the squash and zucchini on the other baking sheet and coat with a little oil, salt, and pepper. If you want caramelized squash and zucchini, you will need to cook them separately from the peppers, as they create a lot of steam as they cook. I cook them together for time and ease.

2. Roast the squash for 30 minutes to an hour, and the peppers for an hour. The peppers should be blistered on top and the flesh soft.

3. Remove the vegetables from the oven and cover the peppers with a kitchen towel to sweat. This will make it easier to peel their skins off.

4. When the peppers are cooled, use your hands to peel off the skins, discarding them along with the cores and seeds. Tear the peppers into rough strips and set aside.

5. **To make the béchamel,** melt the butter in a large saucepan over medium-low heat, then whisk in the cornstarch. Cook for a minute or two, then add the milk, whisking at semi-regular intervals until the mixture starts to thicken. Once it reaches your desired thickness, add in the Parmesan and whisk to combine.

6. Stir in the mozzarella until the mixture becomes a delicious, melty, and stringy sauce. Season with salt and the nutmeg, if using, and remove from the heat.

7. **To finish the lasagna,** preheat the oven to 350°F (180°C), if it isn't already on.

8. Cover the bottom of a 9 × 13-inch (23 × 33 cm) baking dish with a layer of lasagna noodles.

9. Add half of the Bolognese, ensuring you've got even coverage. Add the roasted squash and zucchini, topped with half of the béchamel. Spread it with a spoon as best you can, making sure you get it to the edges of the dish.

10. Next up, add the spinach and basil layer. Now, another layer of lasagna sheets, topped with the roasted pepper strips, then the final layer of Bolognese. Finally, gently spread the remaining béchamel over the top, trying not to disturb the Bolognese.

11. Place the baking dish on a baking sheet to catch any spills and bake for 30 to 40 minutes, until the top is beautiful and brown. Remove from the oven. Slice into six or eight large pieces and serve.

Note: You can wilt and drain the spinach and basil if you'd like—this will remove a little extra moisture from the lasagna.

FODMAP-Friendly Pesto

MAKES 1 CUP
(250 G)

In a past life, I was a strong (inadvertent pun) advocate of using a minimum of six garlic cloves in a single batch of pesto. It has taken me a long time to accept this FODMAP-friendly version as a suitable replacement, but we're finally in a good place. I like to mix it up depending on what I have on hand: Using walnuts makes a slightly bitter but cost-effective pesto, as does arugula.

1 cup (125 g) roughly chopped pine nuts or walnuts
1 large bunch basil (leaves and stems)
1 cup (100 g) finely grated vegetarian Parmesan
Juice of 1 lemon
¼ to ½ cup (60 to 125 ml) extra virgin olive oil (see Note)
Fine salt

1. Combine the pine nuts and basil in a food processor and blend well.
2. Add the Parmesan, lemon juice, and oil and blend again, adding a little more oil, if needed.
3. Add salt to taste and blend until you have reached a pesto consistency.
4. Transfer to an airtight container and cover the pesto with a layer of oil—this seals it and stops it from spoiling too quickly. Store in the fridge and use within a week.

Note: You can experiment with the nut and oil quantities that work for you. I like a good walnut pesto, but I also add an additional ¼ cup (60 ml) of olive oil to account for the comparative dryness of walnuts. You can also use garlic-infused olive oil to impart a garlic taste without unpleasant side effects.

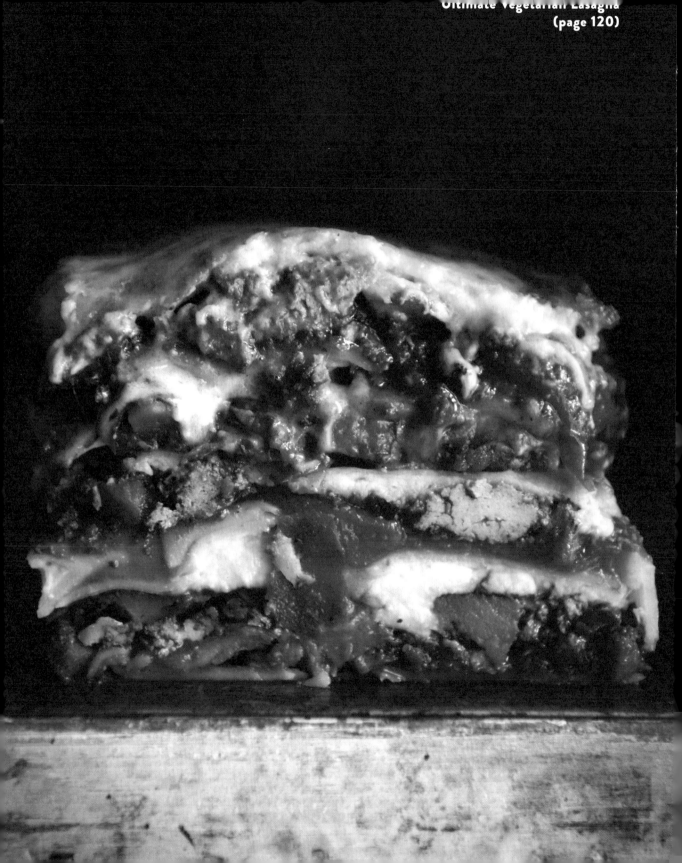

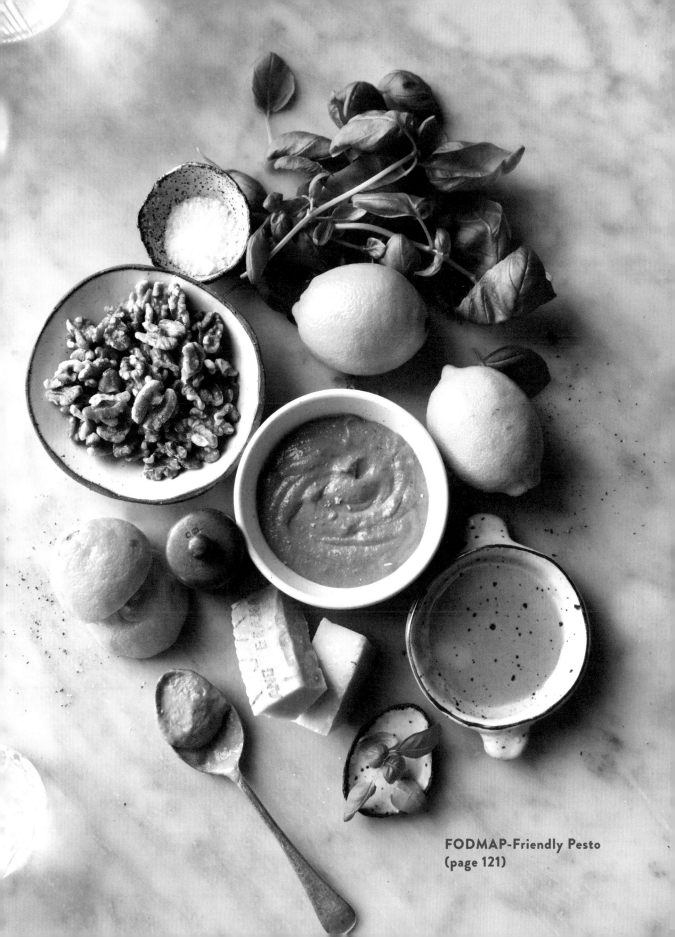

FODMAP-Friendly Pesto
(page 121)

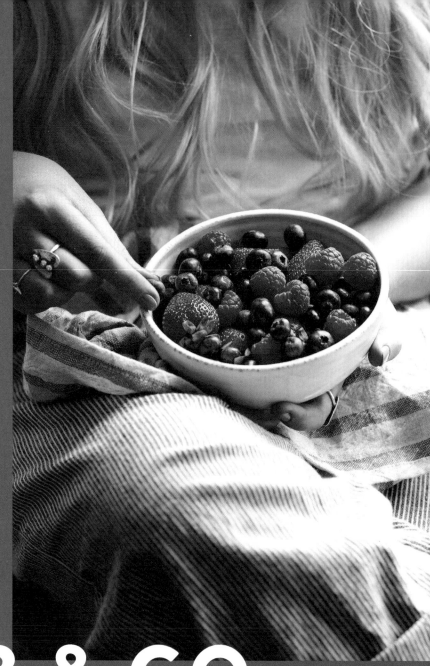

GRAB & GO
BAKING

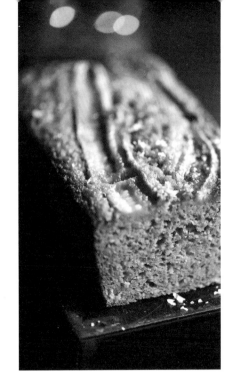

As someone who works predominantly from home, I underestimated the importance of grab-and-go foods until I once forgot to bring a fork for a chopped salad lunch while out and about.

Truth be told, the vast majority of easy, portable snacks available are not so easy on the digestively challenged. Granola bars are laden with dried fruit, salad bars are jammed with onion, and sandwiches are, well, sandwiches.

So, this chapter contains an offering of baked goods that are both easy to transport and easy on the digestive system. This seems like as good a time as any to toot my own horn and write that they're oft easy on the eye, too.

Whether you're after sweet or savory, grab-and-go baking has got your back. And if you're the type of person who carries a stash of chocolate chip cookies around—call me.

Granola Bars

MAKES 8 BARS

Now that everyone is obsessed with Medjool dates, we are inundated with "healthy" granola bars, "sweetened naturally" with the fruits of a small Medjool date tree. This is of no more use to me than the conventional, full-of-sugar variety, so I decided to make my own. Not a single date tree was harmed in the making of these, either. You can decorate your bars with your topping of choice after the two-hour setting time is up, or the next day, if you're leaving them overnight.

1 cup (100 g) gluten-free rolled oats
¼ cup (30 g) macadamia nuts (or preferred low-FODMAP nut)
¼ cup (25 g) pecans (or preferred low-FODMAP nut)
¼ cup (40 g) pepitas
¼ cup (35 g) sunflower seeds
½ cup (160 g) brown rice syrup
¼ cup (60 ml) melted coconut oil
Seeds from 7 cardamom pods, husks discarded
1 teaspoon ground cinnamon
1 teaspoon ground nutmeg
1 teaspoon vanilla bean paste or extract
Pinch of sea salt
¼ cup (30 g) cacao nibs
1 tablespoon chia seeds
1 tablespoon flaxseeds
Neutral oil spray

1. Preheat the oven to 350°F (180°C). Line a baking sheet with parchment paper and spread the oats, nuts, and seeds over it, mixing roughly with your hands. Bake in the oven for 10 minutes. Give the mixture a stir to help distribute heat and browning, then return to the oven for another 10 minutes.

2. Remove the baking sheet from the oven and allow to cool slightly. Transfer to a food processor and pulse—I do four pulses, but this will depend on the strength of your machine. A combination of nut chunks and nut meal is great.

3. In a small saucepan over low heat, combine the rice syrup, oil, spices, vanilla, and salt and cook until everything is combined and fragrant. Turn the heat off and stir in the nut and oat mixture and the cacao nibs to coat everything evenly, then add the chia seeds and flaxseeds.

4. Spray a square baking pan lightly with oil and then line it with beeswax or plastic wrap—enough that there are overhanging edges, with which you can pull the granola bars out later. Spoon the oat mixture into one half of the pan and use your hand to press it down extremely firmly. It will be firm enough to hold its shape despite only filling half the pan.

5. Place in the fridge for at least 2 hours to set (overnight is ideal). Store in the fridge and eat within a week.

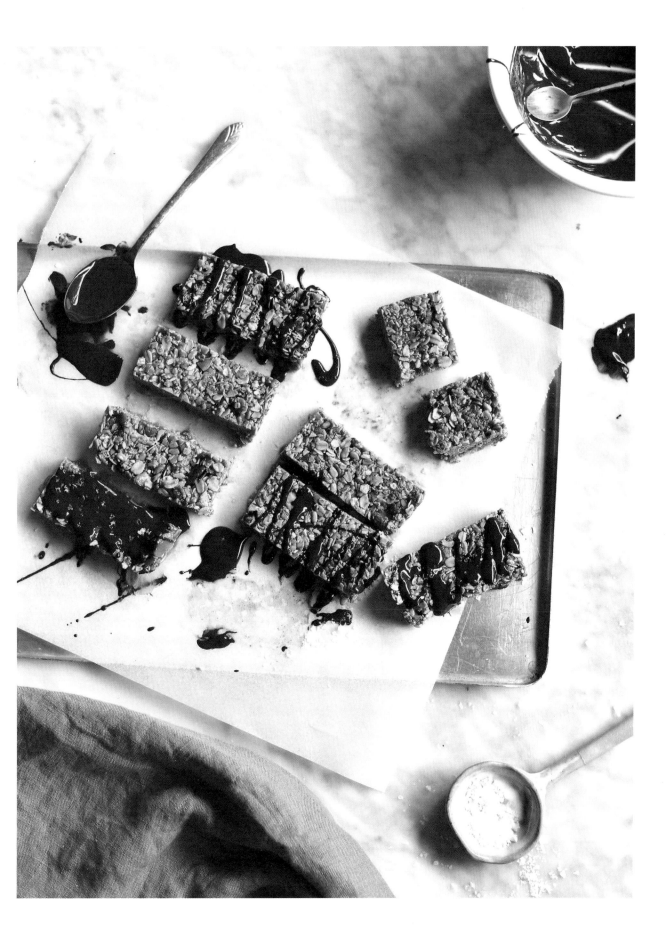

Savory Trail Mix

MAKES ENOUGH
FOR A 24-OUNCE
(750 ML) JAR

Brand me a heretic, but I'm calling it: Chocolate chips are better in savory trail mixes than sweet ones. In the absence of dried fruit, they add a familiar but interesting pop of sweetness, and they pair perfectly with smoky chile flavors. You can play around with the nuts and ratios, or up the quantities of seeds for a nut-free trail mix. You can also omit the chocolate chips if you're not ready to have your life changed. Your call.

½ cup (50 g) walnuts

½ cup (80 g) peanuts

1 cup (160 g) pepitas

1 cup (150 g) sunflower seeds

½ cup (40 g) shredded coconut

1 egg white, thoroughly whisked

1 tablespoon plus 1 teaspoon coconut sugar or light brown sugar

1 heaping teaspoon sea salt

2 teaspoons garam masala

2 teaspoons smoked paprika

1 teaspoon pumpkin pie spice

½ to 1 teaspoon red pepper flakes

½ cup (75 g) dark chocolate chips

1. Preheat the oven to 325°F (160°C). Line a large baking sheet with parchment paper.
2. In a large bowl, mix together the nuts, seeds, and coconut.
3. In a small bowl, combine the egg white, sugar, salt, and spices and whisk together. Pour this spicy mixture over the nut mixture and stir well to combine.
4. Spread out the nut mixture evenly on the baking sheet (use two, if necessary). Bake in the oven for 10 to 15 minutes. Stir to encourage even browning and continue baking for an additional 10 minutes or so, until browned to your liking.
5. Remove from the oven and allow to cool for 10 to 15 minutes, then add the chocolate chips. Don't panic if they melt—they'll grab onto the nuts around them and create chocolatey nut clusters.
6. Allow the mix to cool completely before transferring to an airtight container.

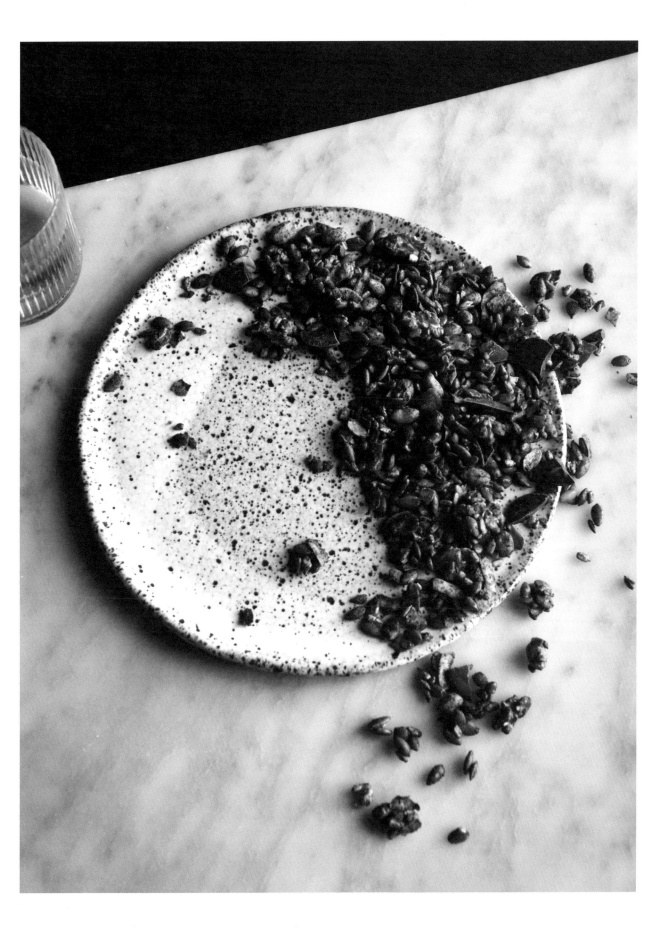

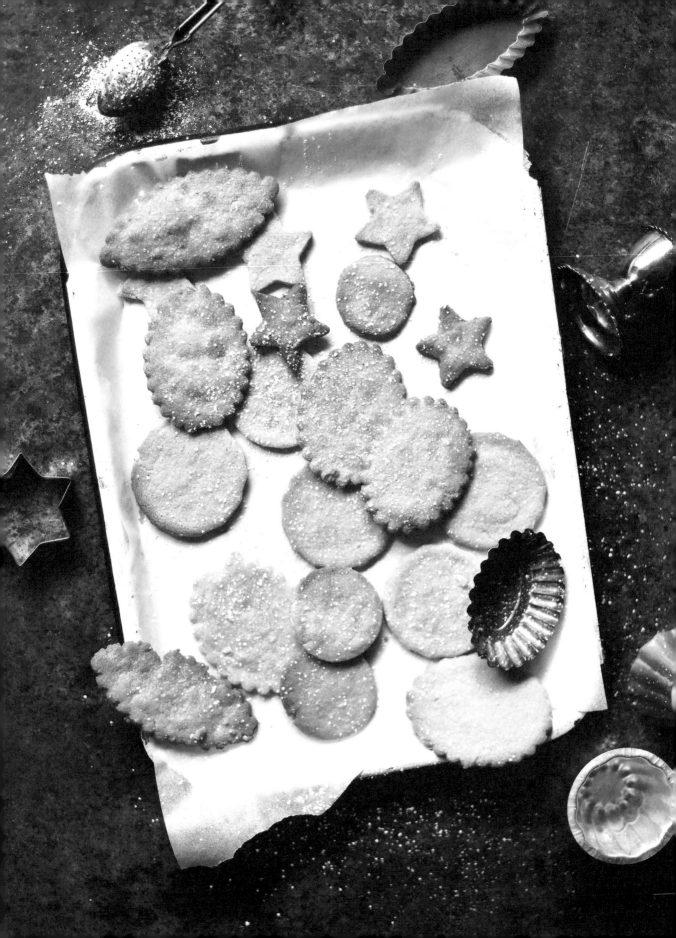

Grain-Free Shortbread Biscuits

MAKES ABOUT
12 SHORTBREADS

Although the vast majority of my childhood culinary memories involve me being sheepishly caught eating other people's food (the neighbor's cat's, strangers' at Kmart, etc.), another standout is making shortbread with my grandma. While my mum openly admits that she used to beat egg whites in the cupboard in the hope we kids wouldn't hear and ask to help, my grandma was saintly patient as I no doubt made a mockery of the shortbread process. It's only fitting to include a recipe in full credit to someone who has had such a big impact on my love of cooking.

1½ cups (150 g) almond meal (see Note)

7 tablespoons (100 g) butter, at room temperature

½ cup (60 g) tapioca flour, plus extra for dusting

1 teaspoon vanilla bean paste or extract

¼ cup (30 g) light brown sugar, not packed

1. Preheat the oven to 350°F (180°C) and line a baking sheet with parchment paper.
2. Combine all the ingredients in a food processor and blitz until a dough has formed. Gather the dough up, wrap it in beeswax or plastic wrap, and transfer to the fridge for around 30 minutes.
3. Sprinkle a sheet of parchment paper with tapioca flour, place the shortbread dough on top, and dust with more flour. Lay a second sheet of parchment paper on top and use a rolling pin to roll the dough out into a layer around ¾ inch (2 cm) thick. (Using lightly floured parchment paper is the easiest way to roll out gluten-free dough without using an ungodly amount of dusting flour.)
4. Use cookie cutters of your choosing to create the shortbread shapes and gently place these onto the baking sheet.
5. Bake the shortbread in the oven for 8 to 10 minutes, until the biscuits are firm and slightly browned. Allow them to cool slightly before consuming—they firm up as they cool. Store in an airtight container for up to a week.

Note: Almond meal is considered FODMAP friendly in servings of ¼ cup (25 g) or less, which is something to keep in mind when you're "evening off" the dough.

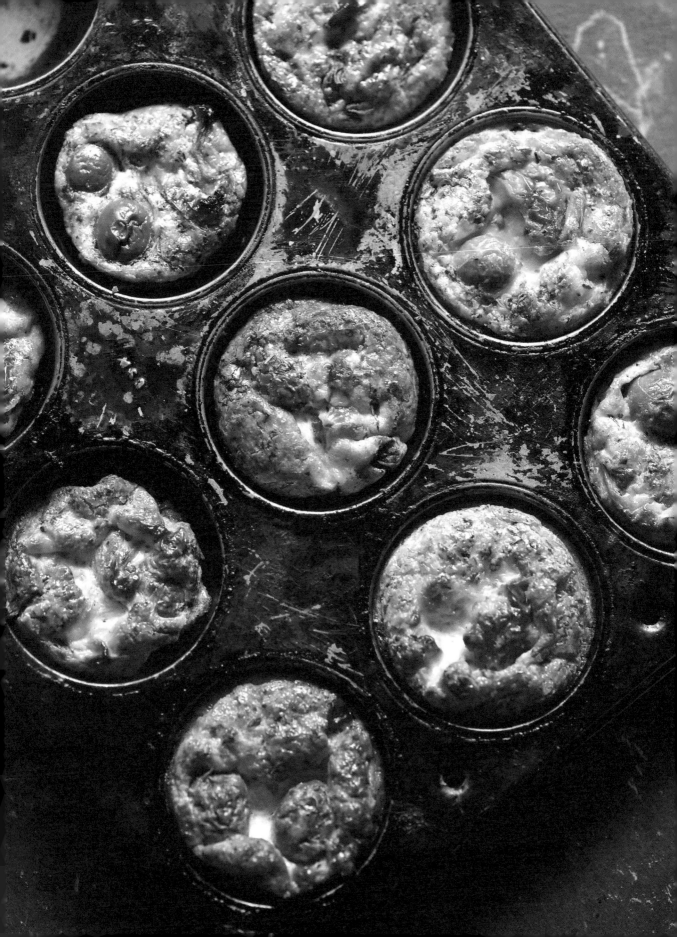

Mini Mediterranean Frittatas

MAKES 8 OR 9
MINI FRITTATAS

I have to admit I've become a bit complacent about how lucky I am to eat a cooked breakfast every morning, as one does when working from home. I don't have to choose between extra sleep and hot food because my boss (me) is a bit too laissez-faire for early starts. That said, the memory of making smoothies the night before my daily work commute (I love food, but I love sleep more) is all too vivid, hence these little frittatas. They are as close as you can get to a full breakfast when you have about five minutes before you need to run out the door.

6 eggs
½ cup (125 ml) milk of your choice
½ cup (50 g) finely grated vegetarian Parmesan
Pinch of dried oregano or ground nutmeg, or both
Good pinch of fine salt
Good pinch of cracked black pepper
½ cup (85 g) Sicilian (Castelvetrano) olives, pitted
½ cup (25 g) sun-dried tomatoes, roughly chopped
Handful of basil leaves, finely chopped

1. Preheat the oven to 350°F (180°C). Grease 9 cups of a 12-cup silicone muffin pan.
2. In a large bowl, whisk together the eggs, milk, Parmesan, oregano and/or nutmeg, and salt and pepper, until well combined.
3. Add the olives, half of the tomatoes, and the basil leaves and stir well.
4. Divide the mixture evenly between 8 or 9 of the muffin cups. Scatter the rest of the tomatoes over the top of the frittatas and gently push them down. Bake in the oven for around 15 minutes, until the frittatas are golden on top and set.
5. Remove from the oven. Allow to cool completely and then keep in an airtight container in the fridge for about 2 to 3 days.

Banana Bread

If you're wondering why I decided to tip my banana bread on its side to pour chocolate over it: I've asked myself the same question. While we're collectively philosophizing, here are the main selling points of this banana bread: It is gluten-free, vegan, and FODMAP friendly. Use bananas that lean toward the unripe end of the scale, if bananas are a trigger for you. Also, note that at the time of print, unripe bananas are considered FODMAP friendly in 3½-ounce (100 g) servings. Restrict yourself to less than a third of the loaf per sitting and you'll be dandy. I call for blueberries as an add-in here, but you could mix in anything you like—chocolate, nuts, whatever. Just make sure it's vegan if it needs to be.

1 cup (130 g) fine white rice flour
¾ cup (75 g) tapioca flour
1½ teaspoons baking powder
1 teaspoon ground cinnamon
1 teaspoon ground nutmeg
1⅓ cups (300 g) mashed bananas (about 3 frozen and thawed or fresh; see Note)
½ cup (120 ml) pure maple syrup
⅓ cup (80 ml) milk of your choice (I used soy milk)
⅓ cup (80 ml) olive oil, or your preferred oil
1 to 2 tablespoons coconut sugar (optional)
1 teaspoon sea salt flakes
2 teaspoons vanilla bean paste or extract
Handful of blueberries (optional)

1. Preheat the oven to 350°F (180°C).
2. In a large mixing bowl, combine the flours, baking powder, and spices.
3. Place the mashed banana in a medium mixing bowl and then add the remaining ingredients, except for the blueberries.
4. Mix the wet ingredients into the dry, stirring to incorporate. Fold in the blueberries (or other add-ins), if using.
5. Pour the mixture into a silicone loaf pan placed on a baking sheet. This makes it easier to keep even and steady.
6. Bake for around 40 minutes, or until the top is perfectly golden. If a skewer doesn't come out clean, cover with foil and continue to bake for another 10 to 15 minutes, until cooked through. Allow to cool a little in the loaf pan before transferring to a wire rack to cool completely before serving or storing.

Note: To use frozen, peeled bananas, place them on a lined baking sheet to defrost as the oven heats. They don't need to be cooked, just thoroughly defrosted. Then, transfer the pieces, along with the juice, to a bowl and mash with a fork.

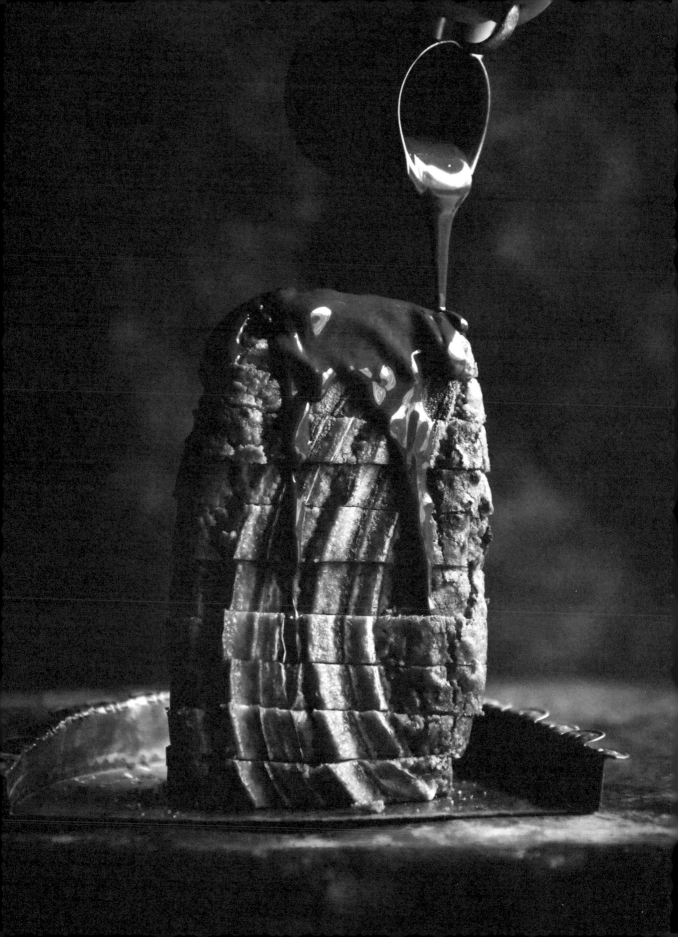

Streusel Muffins

It's been a long time since I've had a café muffin, but this is what I imagine they'd taste like—sans the unbearable sweetness and ten-person serving size. These are gluten-free, nut-free, and dairy-free, and you can experiment with flavorings, toppings, and sugars as you see fit.

Muffins

¾ cup (150 g) plain coconut yogurt

¾ cup (180 ml) almond milk

1 tablespoon apple cider vinegar or lemon juice

¾ cup (100 g) fine brown rice flour

¼ cup (35 g) quinoa flour

¼ cup (30 g) tapioca flour

½ cup (110 g) superfine baker's or caster sugar

2 tablespoons plus 2 teaspoons light brown or coconut sugar

1 tablespoon pumpkin pie spice

2 teaspoons ground nutmeg

1 teaspoon baking powder

½ teaspoon baking soda

2 eggs

½ cup (60 to 80 g) berries of choice, plus extra to top (fresh are preferable as frozen will add extra water content)

Streusel topping (optional)

2½ tablespoons toasted gluten-free rolled oats (toast in a dry pan or the oven)

2 teaspoons light brown sugar

2 teaspoons coconut butter or coconut oil

Pinch of ground nutmeg

1. **To make the muffins,** preheat the oven to 350°F (180°C) and grease 10 cups of a 12-cup silicone muffin pan.

2. In a large bowl, combine the yogurt, milk, and vinegar. Stir to combine, then allow to sit for 10 minutes to form a buttermilk of sorts.

3. In a separate large bowl, combine the dry ingredients and mix well.

4. Pour the "buttermilk" into the bowl of dry ingredients and add the eggs, stirring well to form a batter. Once thoroughly combined, fold in the berries to gently distribute them through the mixture.

5. **To make the streusel topping,** if using, rub the oats, sugar, butter, and nutmeg together with your hands until the oats are sticky and coated.

6. **To finish,** pour the batter into the prepared muffin pan and top with a sprinkle of streusel and the additional berries. Bake in the oven for 25 to 30 minutes, until the tops of the muffins are browned and firm.

7. Cool for a minute or so, then carefully remove them from the pan and place them on a wire rack to cool before eating. They keep well in an airtight container in the fridge for a couple of days.

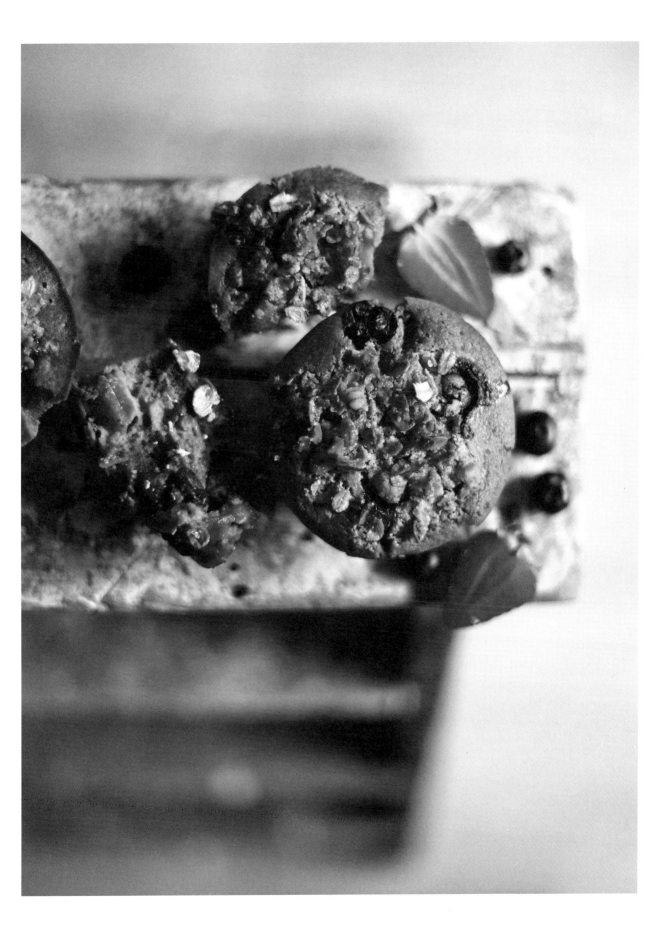

Pumpkin, Sage, Feta, and Pine Nut Muffins

MAKES 8 MUFFINS

If these needed an alternate name, I'd call them "A test of how many delicious things you can stuff into a single mouthful of muffin." They are jam-packed, but the inclusion of psyllium husk keeps them from falling to pieces. If psyllium husk could do the same for me, that would be much appreciated.

3 eggs

1 tablespoon psyllium husk

4 cups (500 g) peeled, cubed pumpkin or other winter squash, half steamed and the other half roasted

½ cup (50 g) almond meal

½ cup (65 g) fine brown rice flour

¼ cup (35 g) quinoa flour

¼ cup (30 g) tapioca flour

2 teaspoons baking powder

7 tablespoons (100 g) butter

2 tablespoons plus 2 teaspoons milk of your choice

½ cup (80 g) pine nuts

5 or 6 large sage leaves, finely sliced

⅔ cup (100 g) crumbled feta (vegan cheese also works, if you'd like to lower the lactose content)

2 teaspoons apple cider vinegar

1. Preheat the oven to 350°F (180°C) and grease 8 cups of a 12-cup silicone muffin pan.
2. Whisk together the eggs and psyllium husk and set aside to gel. It will become the glue that holds the muffins together.
3. In a food processor, combine the steamed pumpkin, almond meal, flours, baking powder, butter, and milk, and process until an orange batter forms. Once the psyllium has gelled, add it to the batter and pulse a few times to combine.
4. You can transfer the batter to another bowl or continue working in the food processor, one-pot-wonder style. Either way, add the remaining ingredients and stir gently to combine.
5. Divide the mixture evenly between the muffin cups and bake in the oven for 25 to 30 minutes, until the muffins are beautifully browned on top.
6. Allow to cool slightly before gently running a knife around each muffin and popping them out.
7. Serve or cool completely to store in an airtight container, and eat within 2 to 3 days.

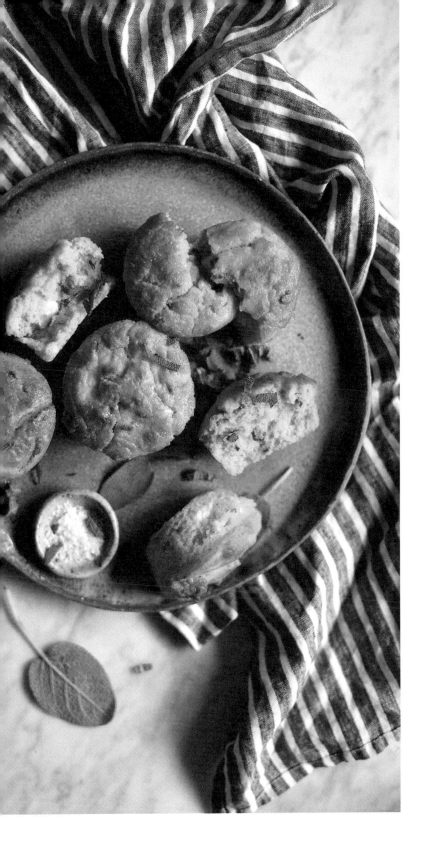
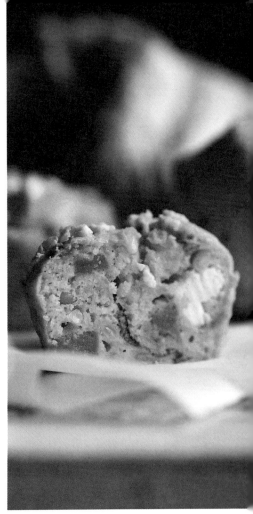

Hot Cross Buns

MAKES 12 TO 14 BUNS

Say hello to your breakfast from early March until at least the end of April. I've used chocolate chips instead of dried fruit and white chocolate for crossing them.

Dough

2 cups (260 g) fine white rice flour

1 cup (120 g) tapioca flour

1 tablespoon ground cinnamon

1 tablespoon ground nutmeg

2 teaspoons pumpkin pie spice

2 teaspoons baking powder

¾ cup (90 g) plus 1 teaspoon light brown sugar, not packed

One ¼-ounce (7 g) packet active dry yeast

¾ cup (180 ml) milk of your choice, warmed

3 eggs

¼ cup (20 g) psyllium husk

½ cup (125 ml) warm water

½ cup (110 g) butter, melted

1 teaspoon vanilla bean paste or extract

1 tablespoon olive oil

½ cup (75 g) dark chocolate chips

To finish

1 egg, lightly beaten, for egg wash

1 ounce (30 g) white chocolate, melted (optional)

1. **To make the dough,** combine the flours, spices, baking powder, and ¾ cup of the sugar in a large bowl.

2. In another bowl, combine the yeast, milk, and the remaining teaspoon of sugar and allow to sit for 15 to 20 minutes, until the surface is bubbly and expanded. If your yeast doesn't form bubbles in this time, it won't give your baking any lift so discard it and start again.

3. While the yeast is activating, whisk the eggs in a small bowl and add the psyllium husk. Continue to whisk until the mixture starts to stiffen and form a blob. Add the warm water, stir to incorporate, and then add the butter and vanilla. Stir well and allow to sit for 15 to 20 minutes, until the mixture is a firm, cohesive lump. Don't panic or be weirded out—this "lump" mimics the elastic nature of gluten and will help to ensure your buns don't taste like cardboard. Hooray, lump!

4. Once the yeast has risen and the psyllium husk blob has formed, stir both of these into the flour mixture, followed by the oil. Knead until the dough forms a ball and then add the chocolate chips. Using lightly greased hands, divide the mixture into small buns and place them on a baking sheet lined with parchment paper. They will rise a little, so give them a bit of room.

5. Cover the buns with a kitchen towel and allow to rise for an hour in a warm, draft-free place. (I set mine on the oven while I'm cooking other things.) If you're not cooking, preheat the oven to 350°F (180°C) 10 minutes before the buns have finished rising.

6. **To finish,** gently paint the egg wash over each of the buns and bake in the oven for 15 to 20 minutes, until nicely browned. Remove from the oven. If you're crossing them with the white chocolate, cool them completely before piping on with a piping bag. These are best eaten right away but are still great warmed or toasted for 3 to 4 days after baking, with a generous slather of butter.

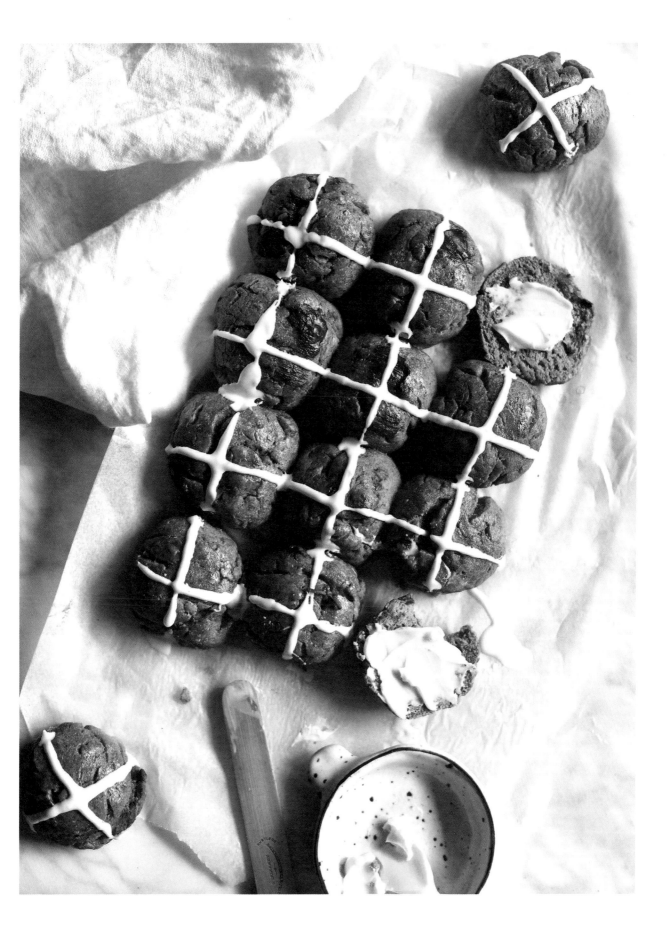

Vegan Chocolate Chip Cookies

MAKES 8 TO 10
MEDIUM COOKIES

If there was a blank page in this book for every time I tested these cookies, there would be more than sixty-five blank pages. Vegan *and* gluten-free cookies are a fine art, and I'd highly recommend reading my extensive notes on them on my website. Main takeaways: Use a high-fat-percentage vegan butter, weigh all your ingredients instead of using the volume measures, and don't skip the salt. Go read my notes on them. Let me save you all those pages of heartbreak.

⅓ cup (75 g) cold vegan butter (needs at least 9 g fat per tablespoon)

⅓ cup plus 1 tablespoon (50 g) light brown sugar, not packed

2 tablespoons plus 2 teaspoons superfine baker's or caster sugar

1 teaspoon vanilla extract

½ cup plus 2 teaspoons (55 g) tapioca flour, plus up to 2½ tablespoons (15 g) more if needed

¼ cup (30 g) brown rice flour (make sure it's finely milled)

1 teaspoon baking powder

¼ teaspoon fine salt

2 teaspoons cold soy milk

1¾ to 3½ ounces (50 to 100 g) vegan chocolate (I used Lindt dark)

Sea salt flakes, to finish

1. **The first day:** Measure out the butter, straight from the fridge, and the sugars and place them in the bowl of your kitchen mixer. (You can probably do this with a hand mixer, but Mama ain't got time to make sixty cookies that way.)

2. Add the vanilla and then cream for 1 minute on a high speed. Use a spatula to wipe down the bowl edges, making sure there's no rogue butter or sugar there. Cream for another minute. The mixture should look like a light-colored cookie batter, and the whisk should leave tracks. Place in the fridge to chill.

3. With a clean, dry whisk, combine the flours, baking powder, and salt in a small bowl.

4. Remove the butter mixture from the fridge and mix in the soy milk, until the edges pull away from the bowl.

5. Add the flour mixture, ensuring you get every little bit. Use a spoon to mix and mix and mix until the cookie dough comes together and is just too wet to handle.

6. Cover the cookie dough and refrigerate overnight.

7. **The next day:** Preheat the oven to 350°F (180°C). If you like a fatter cookie, you can cook them at 325°F (160°C). Place the baking sheet in the freezer for 10 minutes before use to help stop excess cookie spread.

8. Chop the chocolate and stir into the cookie dough.

9. Bake one cookie solo first, just to check that it comes out exactly how you want it. Spoon 1 tablespoon of the dough onto the baking sheet (shaggy edges are fine) and bake for 10 minutes. (Chill the rest of the dough while you bake.) Remove and gently bang the baking sheet on the oven rack to release the gas. Bake for longer if it needs browning, but only 1 or 2 minutes, so it's still gooey inside. Let sit on the baking sheet for a minute, then transfer to a cool surface and rest 5 minutes before testing. (Don't pick them up before this time—they are molten sugar without an egg to bind and will need time to cool.)

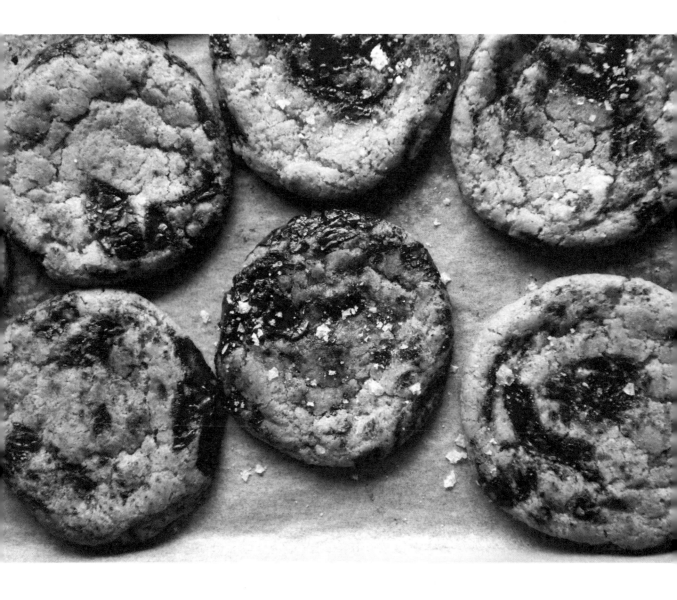

10. If the cookie is too flat, make sure you didn't spoon too much on or neglect to follow any previous instructions, otherwise add 2 teaspoons (5 g) extra tapioca flour. To address a puffy cookie with no spread, add 1 extra teaspoon soy milk.

11. If all systems are go, place four 1-tablespoon blobs of the dough evenly across the cooled baking sheet and bake 10 to 12 minutes, remembering to bang out the gas and to cool them before handling or eating.

Banana, Peanut Butter, Chocolate, and Coconut Muffins

MAKES 7 TO
8 MUFFINS

This one is for the FODMAP, gluten-free vegans—you must be going through it, because I certainly was while I was developing this recipe. If you don't need the muffins to be vegan, you can use regular chocolate, but otherwise, find a brand of vegan chocolate with as few weird additives as possible.

½ cup (55 g) cocoa powder

¼ cup (60 ml) melted coconut oil

1 banana, mashed

¾ cup (180 ml) almond milk

½ cup (110 g) light brown sugar, packed

¼ cup (60 ml) maple syrup

¼ cup (50 g) coconut yogurt

2 tablespoons plus 2 teaspoons natural peanut butter

Pinch of sea salt, plus extra for serving

1 teaspoon baking powder

½ teaspoon baking soda

2 teaspoons vinegar

1 cup (130 g) fine rice flour

1¾ ounces (50 g) vegan chocolate, broken into small chunks

1. Preheat the oven to 350°F (180°C) and grease 8 cups of a 12-cup silicone muffin pan.

2. In a large bowl, whisk together the cocoa and coconut oil, ensuring there are no lumps. Add the banana, milk, sugar, maple syrup, yogurt, peanut butter, and salt and continue to whisk until combined.

3. Stir in the baking powder and baking soda, then the vinegar. Finally, add the flour and mix until a batter forms.

4. Pour the batter into the greased muffin cups and gently press a few chunks of chocolate into the top of each muffin. Bake for 35 minutes, or until the muffins are firm but springy. Immediately transfer to a wire rack to prevent soggy bottoms (but take care as the muffins will be delicate fresh out of the oven). Sprinkle on a pinch of salt, if you like, to intensify the chocolate flavor.

5. Store in an airtight container and eat within 2 to 3 days.

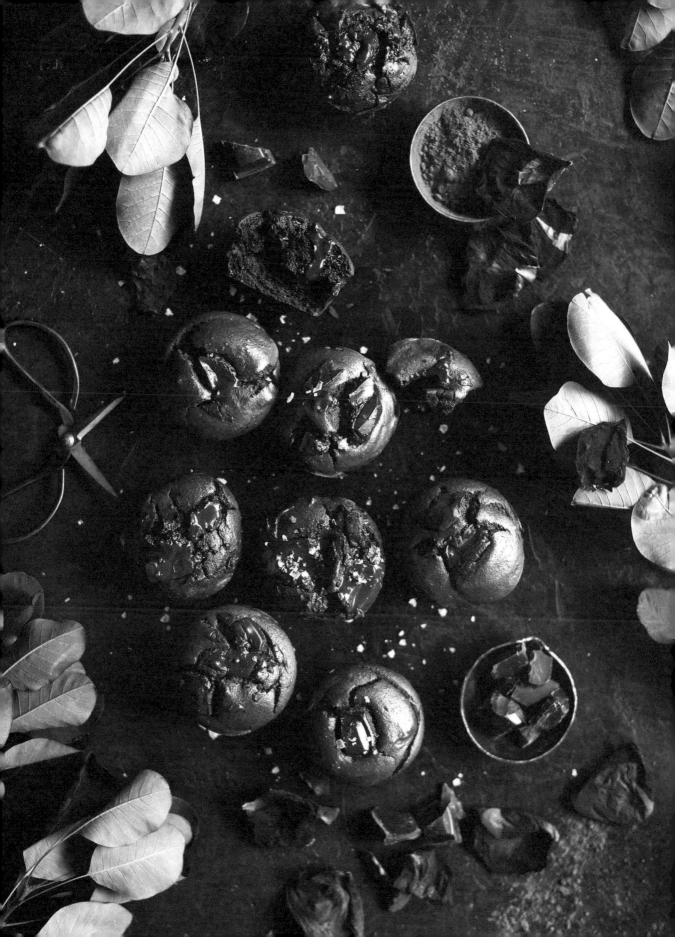

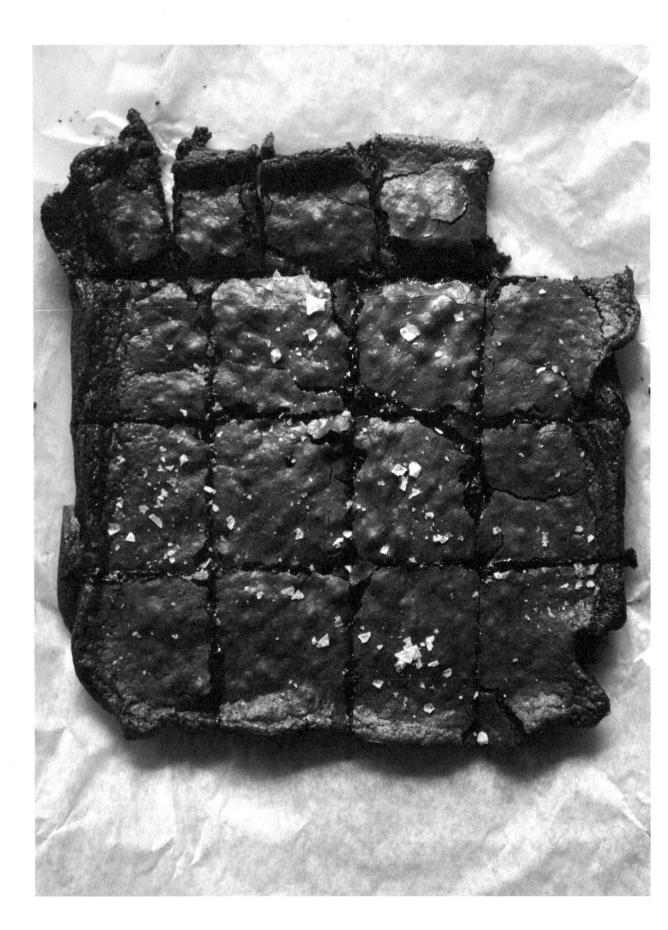

Best-Ever Gluten-Free Chocolate Brownies

MAKES 16 SMALL BROWNIES

Like a total megalomaniac, I have titled these brownies the "best-ever" gluten- and grain-free brownies. I hate to toot my own horn (not really) but they are really *that good*. I have numerous different brownie recipes on my website if you need a nut-free/vegan/brown butter version. These brownies are best made the night before. I also highly recommend keeping these in the fridge—when they're fresh from the oven, they can be hard to eat for their fudginess. I like to sprinkle my brownies with a little extra sea salt, but you do you.

¾ cup (175 g) butter

1 cup (220 g) superfine baker's or caster sugar (or ½ light brown and ½ superfine)

3 large eggs

6 ounces (200 g) dark baking chocolate (I use 70 percent cacao)

2 tablespoons plus 2 teaspoons Dutch-processed cocoa powder

2 teaspoons vanilla bean paste or extract

1 teaspoon sea salt flakes

1 tablespoon freshly brewed espresso

1 tablespoon hot water

¾ to 1 cup (75 to 100 g) almond meal

1. In a small saucepan, melt the butter over low heat, then add the sugar and stir well to combine. Turn the heat off and leave the mixture to cool for 10 minutes or so. If it's too hot, it will cook the eggs.

2. Transfer to a kitchen mixer with a whisk attachment. While beating on a medium speed, add the eggs, one at a time, then continue to beat on a medium speed for 10 minutes. This will help create the meringue-like crackly top.

3. Preheat the oven to 350°F (180°C) and line a lightly oiled 9-inch (23 cm) square baking pan with parchment paper.

4. While the mixture is beating, melt the chocolate using a double boiler, then remove from the heat.

5. Add the cocoa, vanilla, and salt to the chocolate. Pour in the espresso and hot water to "bloom" the cocoa—bring out the depth of the chocolate flavor. Gently stir the mixture until just combined.

6. Turn off the stand mixer and add the chocolate mixture to the bowl. Mix on a low speed until just combined. The batter should be silky, smooth, and medium brown in color.

7. Add the almond meal and stir until just combined. Pour into the prepared pan and bake in the oven for 20 to 35 minutes, depending on how "done" you like your brownies.

8. For best, most delicious results, allow to cool before slicing and eating.

Gingerbread

MAKES 8 TO 10 GINGERBREAD COOKIES

1 cup (225 g) light roasted almond butter (see Note)
½ cup (120 ml) pure maple syrup
1 tablespoon ground ginger
2 teaspoons ground cinnamon
2 teaspoons ground nutmeg
½ teaspoon ground clove
1 teaspoon baking powder
2 teaspoons vanilla bean paste, or 2 more teaspoons maple syrup
Pinch of fine salt

The worst thing about Christmas is the fuss involved in making gluten-free gingerbreads. These are the cheatiest gluten-free gingerbreads in all the lands—no flours, no insanely sticky dough, no worries.

1. Preheat the oven to 350°F (180°C). Lightly grease a sheet of parchment paper and line a baking sheet with a plain piece of parchment.

2. Combine all the ingredients for the cookies together in a medium mixing bowl. Mix until the batter thickens and becomes solid enough to pick up. This might take a little while, 5 minutes or so, and sometimes it helps to have a break from stirring. It will thicken while it rests. (Read the Note on the best almond butter to use to make sure you're not fighting a losing battle.)

3. Lightly oil your hands and transfer the dough onto the oiled parchment. Flatten the dough out using the palm of your hands. The thickness is up to you, but I like a thick gingerbread. Mine are roughly ¼ inch (5 mm) thick—adjust the cooking time if you like yours thicker/thinner.

4. You can begin gently cutting the cookies right away, but I find it easiest to put the flattened dough in the freezer for 15 to 20 minutes. When the dough is cold, it is far less likely to be stretchy and petulant.

5. Place the cookies on the lined baking sheet, leaving some room for spread-age (this depends a little on the almond butter you use). Bake anywhere from 8 to 15 minutes, according to your taste. Baking 8 minutes means chewy on the outside and soft on the inside (in my oven), and 10 or more leans toward a more well-cooked and crunchy bake. Your call.

6. Allow the cookies to completely cool before touching or moving them—they will harden as they cool. Once cooled, store in an airtight container to prevent them from getting soggy. Eat within a few days.

Note: I've had the best luck with supermarket-variety, 100 percent roasted almond butter. It's oily, but not too oily, and mostly smooth. If your almond butter is too thin or oily, you won't be able to bring the mixture together into a moldable dough. If it's too thick or dry, you'll get cracked gingerbreads. So, a middle ground is important. I wouldn't recommend a dark roasted almond butter for this recipe, since it would make the cookies too "well browned" in taste, and would give a definitive almond flavor to them, which we don't really want.

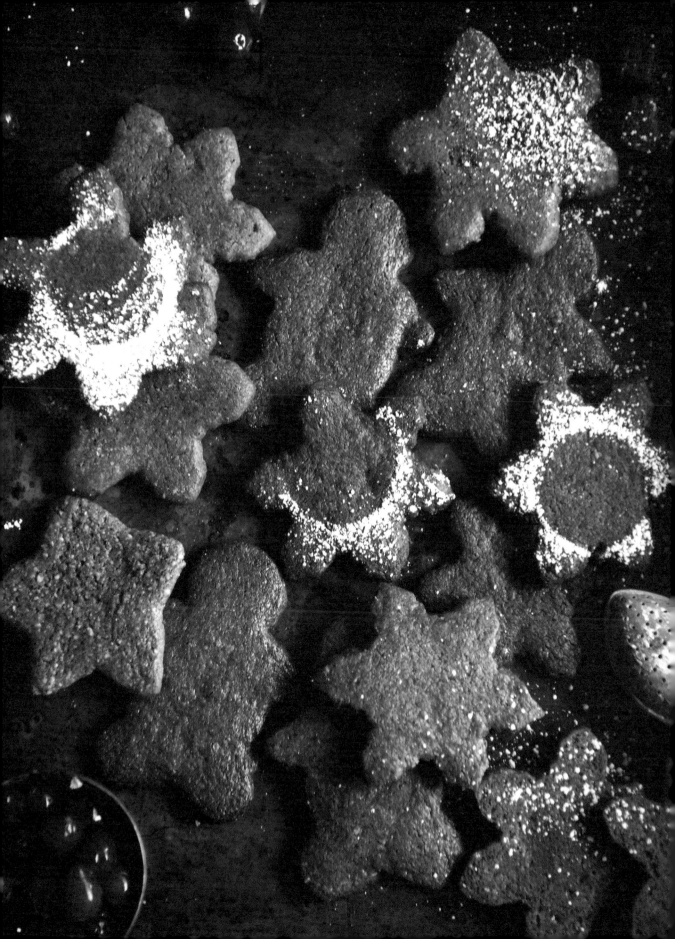

THE SWEET
LIFE

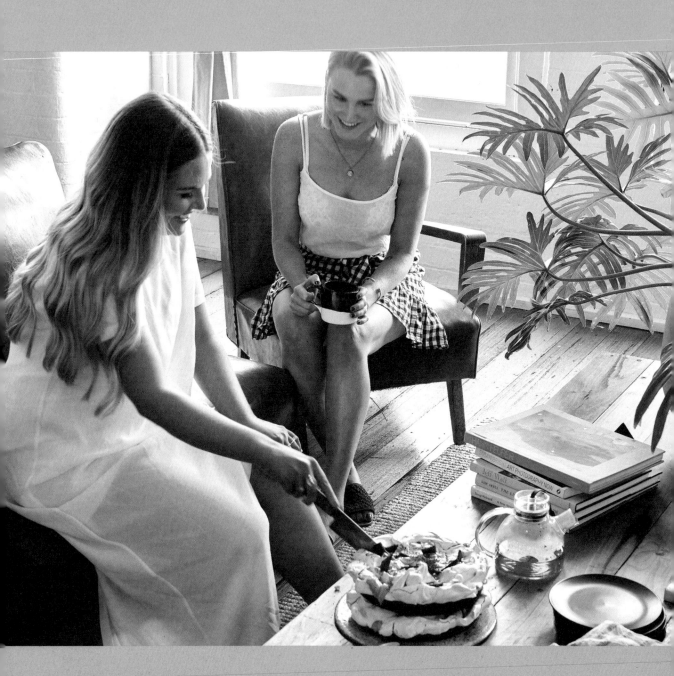

The dessert chapter is always the first part of a cookbook I examine, so naturally, I covertly spread the sweets throughout three-plus chapters of this book.

All life's celebratory moments are best punctuated by sweets, and intolerance-friendly baking can be a fickle friend. I've collated some of my favorite gluten-free desserts here, some of which I've been making (otherwise known as: strongly suggesting my mum make) since I was a teenager.

Cobbler, pumpkin pie, doughnuts, and flourless chocolate cake—the best punctuations are all here.

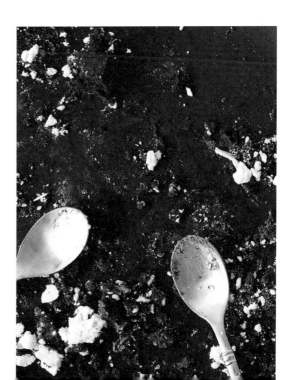

Grain-Free Chocolate Cake

MAKES ONE
9-INCH (23 CM)
CAKE (SERVES 8)

I've been making and asking for this chocolate cake ever since I've been making and asking for cake. I requested it every birthday without fail, long before I learned what gluten was, or that my digestive system would fall in a heap. To keep things exciting (and dare I say, slightly more akin to that infamous chocolate hazelnut spread), you can use hazelnut meal in place of the almond meal. If you're really trying to eliminate butter (as low in lactose and FODMAPs as it is), vegan butter is a great substitute.

13 ounces (375 g) dark chocolate, roughly chopped

1 cup plus 5 tablespoons (300 g) butter or vegan butter, diced

6 eggs

½ cup (110 g) superfine baker's or caster sugar

¼ cup (25 g) almond meal

2½ tablespoons freshly made espresso (optional)

Confectioners' sugar, for dusting (optional)

1. Preheat the oven to 350°F (180°C). Grease a 9-inch (23 cm) springform cake pan and line the bottom with parchment paper.
2. Melt the chocolate and butter together in a heatproof bowl placed over a small pot of water on low heat. Ensure the water doesn't touch the base of the bowl.
3. Separate your eggs carefully and set the egg yolks aside. Whip the egg whites in a clean bowl until they have stiff peaks.
4. Once the chocolate and butter have melted together, take them off the heat and allow to cool slightly.
5. Add the superfine sugar, almond meal, and egg yolks to the chocolate and mix well to combine.
6. Transfer to a large bowl and very gently fold the egg whites into the chocolate. I fold a quarter of the egg whites into the chocolate at a time, to make sure they don't lose their fluffiness—this is what gives the cake height, in the absence of flour. Fold the espresso in now, too, if using.
7. Pour the batter into the prepared pan and bake for 40 minutes.
8. Check with a skewer and continue cooking until the skewer comes out mostly clean. It should take around 50 minutes, depending on your oven. Allow to cool slightly before removing from the pan and slicing. Dust with confections' sugar, if you like.

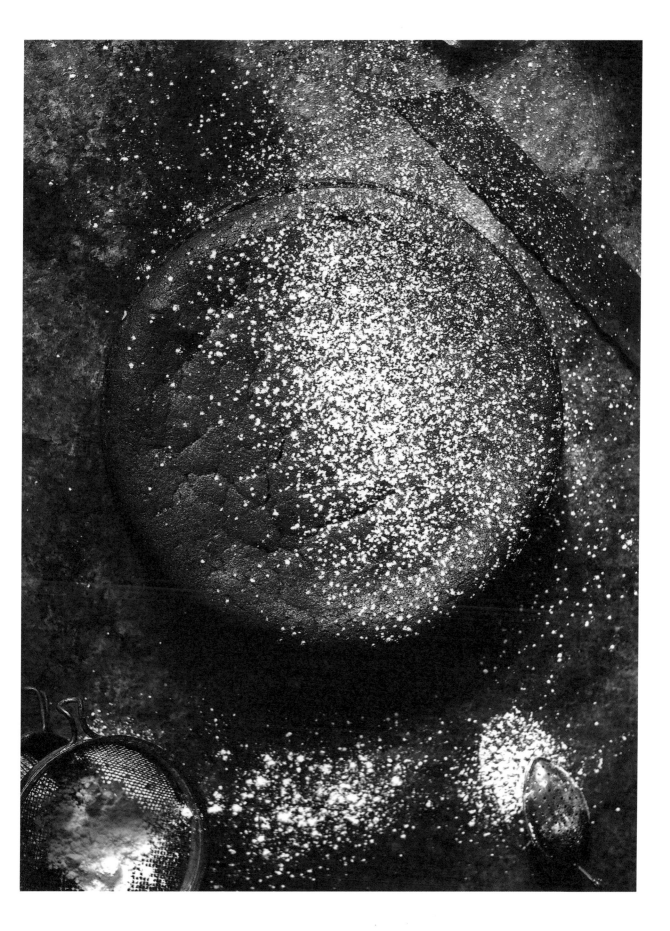

Baked Doughnuts

MAKES 8 TO
10 DONUTS

I'm a purist at heart, and there's no doughnut I prefer more than a cinnamon sugar doughnut. These ones include an undetectable amount of yogurt to keep them *moist* and undetectably gluten-free. Make sure it's plain in flavor and lactose-free if it needs to be.

Doughnuts

7 tablespoons (100 g) butter, melted and slightly cooled, plus more for greasing

1¼ cups (150 g) fine white rice flour

½ cup (50 g) tapioca flour

1½ teaspoons baking powder

¼ teaspoon baking soda

⅓ cup plus 2 tablespoons (100 g) superfine baker's or caster sugar

1 teaspoon ground cinnamon

1 teaspoon ground nutmeg

Pinch of fine salt

¼ cup (60 ml) vegetable oil or other neutral oil

2 extra-large eggs

1 cup (225 g) full-fat lactose-free plain yogurt

1 teaspoon vanilla bean paste or extract

To finish

7 tablespoons (100 g) butter, melted (optional, see Note)

¼ cup (55 g) superfine baker's or caster sugar

½ to 1 teaspoon ground cinnamon

1. **To make the doughnuts,** preheat the oven to 350°F (180°C) and grease a doughnut pan with butter.
2. In a large mixing bowl, combine the flours, baking powder, baking soda, sugar, spices, and salt. Use a whisk to thoroughly combine.
3. Add the butter, oil, yogurt, and eggs to the dry ingredients. Mix thoroughly until there are no dry patches and the batter is uniform in consistency.
4. Transfer the batter into a piping bag or a sandwich bag with a little snip in one of the corners. Pipe the batter into the doughnut pan and repeat until you have used all the batter. Depending on how many doughnut pans you have, you might need to do this in batches.
5. Bake each batch in the oven for 13 to 15 minutes, until slightly golden, risen, and firm. Remove the pan from the oven and allow the doughnuts to rest for a few minutes before gently removing them from the pan. Place on a wire rack to cool.
6. **To finish,** if you've ascertained you need it (see Note), melt the butter in a small saucepan. In a shallow bowl, mix together the sugar and cinnamon to taste.
7. Carefully and quickly dunk each doughnut while still warm in the butter (front and back), and then dip each side in the cinnamon sugar. Return to the wire rack to cool completely.

Note: I find that warm doughnuts often don't need butter to help cinnamon sugar adhere to them. Only use the butter if you've found that the cinnamon sugar isn't sticking. If you're using butter, make sure you dip the doughnuts while they're still warm, as they seem to absorb more butter once cooled.

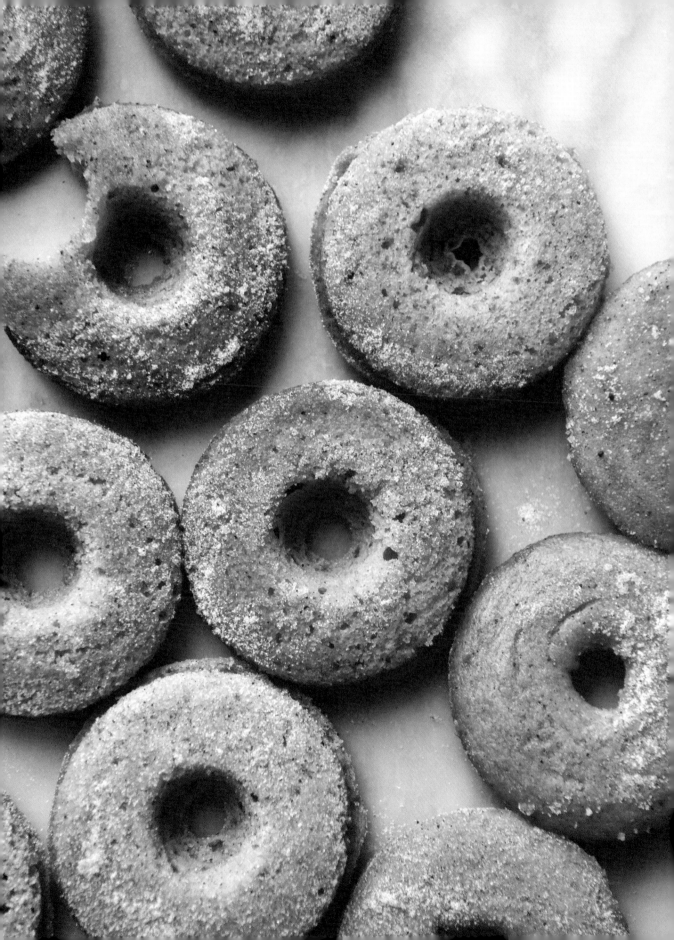

Pavlova with Roasted Lemony Strawberries

SERVES 8 TO 12

I wasn't aware that pavlova could be improved—then I tried lemon-roasted strawberries on one. . . .

Roasted lemony strawberries

9 ounces (250 g; about 1¾ cups) strawberries, hulled and halved

Zest and juice of 1 lemon

1 teaspoon light brown or coconut sugar

Meringue

Olive oil spray

6 egg whites

1½ cups (330 g) superfine baker's or caster sugar

1 teaspoon vanilla bean paste or extract

½ teaspoon white vinegar

1 tablespoon gluten-free cornstarch

To serve (optional)

Coconut yogurt or whipping cream (lactose-free is preferable)

1. **To make the roasted strawberries,** preheat the oven to 350°F (180°C). Line a baking sheet with parchment paper.
2. Combine all the ingredients in a bowl, mix well, and leave to macerate for 10 to 15 minutes.
3. Place the berries on the lined baking sheet and roast in the oven for 10 to 15 minutes, until they are bright red and juicy. Remove from the oven, allow to cool, and then place in the fridge until you need them. (You'll need the roasted berry juice to serve, so don't discard it.)
4. **To make the meringue,** turn the oven up to 400°F (200°C). Spray a large baking sheet with oil and lay a large sheet of parchment paper on top. The oil will stop the paper from sliding around when you spread the meringue.
5. In a very clean bowl, beat the egg whites with an electric mixer on a medium setting, until they form soft peaks.
6. Add half the sugar and continue to beat until combined. Repeat with the remaining sugar and turn the mixer up to a high speed, until the mixture is combined and no grittiness remains.
7. Turn the mixer to a low speed and mix in the vanilla and vinegar for 30 seconds only. Remove the beater(s) and sift in the cornstarch. Gently use a spatula to just fold the cornstarch into the meringue.
8. **To make the pavlova,** use the spatula to gently spread the meringue into an 8-inch (20 cm) disk on the baking sheet. Pop it in the oven and immediately turn the heat down to 250°F (120°C). Bake for 80 to 90 minutes, intermittently checking that the pavlova hasn't gone brown. It should be pale and firm outside but soft inside. Turn off the oven and leave the pavlova inside. Cool completely with the oven door ajar, then layer the strawberries and yogurt, if you're using it, followed by a drizzle of the strawberry juices.

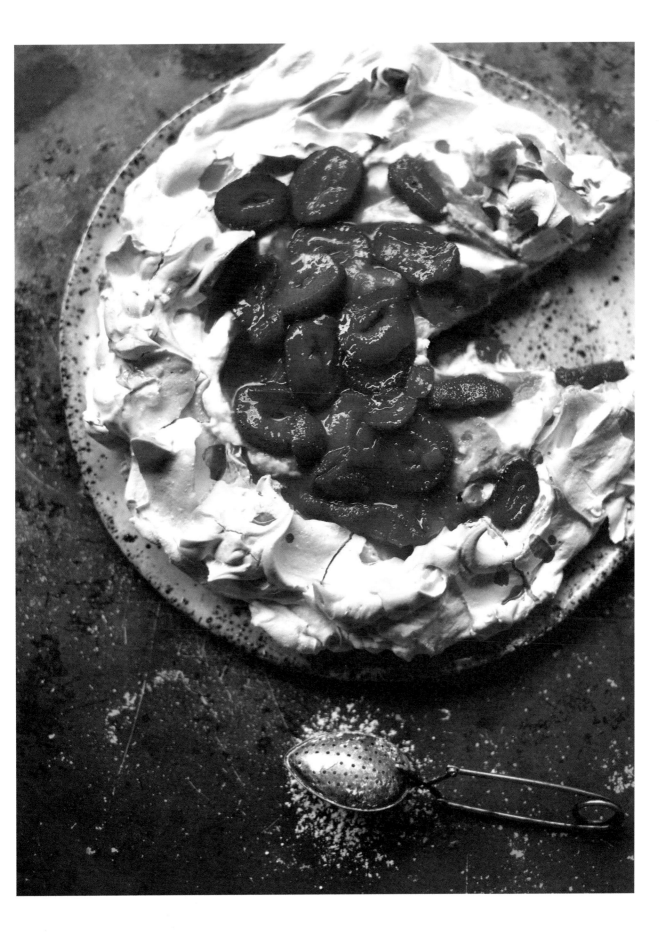

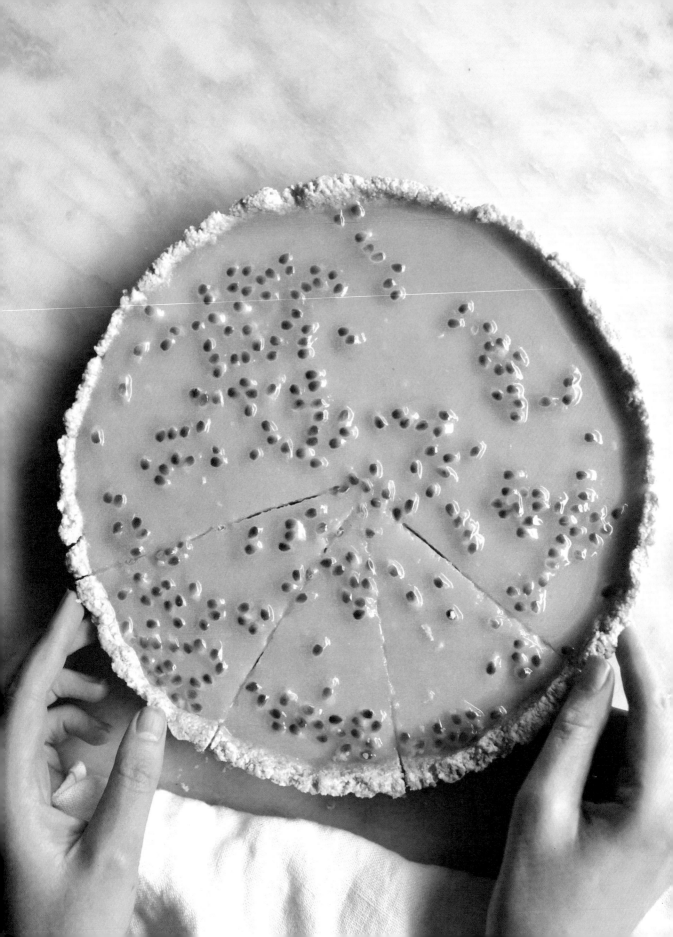

Dairy-Free Lemon Curd Tart with Oat and Coconut Crust

Throughout the recipe-development stage of this book, I was fervently attached to a traditional butter-filled curd for this tart. As a late-stage epiphany, however (apologies to my editor), I attempted a dairy-free version. Although I could easily eat butter by the spoonful, I wouldn't go back to making curd with it, as the lemon is really given a chance to shine. This tart crust is nut-free, but you can use any recipe that fits your dietary requirements. Or, you know, skip the crust entirely and eat the curd with a spoon.

Tart crust

2 cups (200 g) gluten-free rolled oats

½ cup (45 g) desiccated coconut

2 tablespoons plus 2 teaspoons superfine baker's or caster sugar

2 eggs

¼ cup (60 ml) melted coconut oil

Lemon curd

½ cup (110 g) superfine baker's or caster sugar

Zest of 1 lemon

¾ cup (180 ml) freshly squeezed lemon juice

4 eggs plus 1 extra egg yolk

½ cup (125 ml) melted coconut oil (see Note)

1 tablespoon olive oil

To finish

Seeds of 2 passion fruits, or any fruit of your choice (optional)

1. To make the tart crust, place the oats in a food processor and blitz until they form a fine meal. Add the remaining ingredients and process until a wet dough forms. Grease a sheet of beeswax or plastic wrap. Transfer the dough to the plastic, cover, and flatten into a disk. Place in the fridge for 20 minutes to firm up.

2. Preheat the oven to 350°F (180°C) and grease an 8-inch (20 cm) fluted tart pan.

3. Gently press the dough evenly into the pan, guiding it about halfway up the sides. Bake in the oven for 10 to 15 minutes, until lightly golden. Set aside.

4. Meanwhile, to make the lemon curd, use your fingertips to rub the sugar and lemon zest together in a heatproof bowl. Place the bowl over a saucepan of water set over medium heat (making sure the water isn't touching the bottom of the bowl). Add the remaining ingredients and whisk gently for around 10 minutes, until you have a thick, smooth curd that coats the back of a spoon.

5. Pour the curd into the tart crust, gently jiggling the pan to ensure the curd distributes evenly. Bake in the oven for 15 to 20 minutes, until the curd is firm to the touch.

6. Remove from the oven and allow to cool completely before garnishing with the passion fruit seeds (if using), slicing, and serving.

Note: When adding the melted coconut oil to the curd mixture, make sure it's not too hot or it may curdle the eggs.

Salted Caramel Shortbread

SERVES
8 TO 10

In terms of being high maintenance, this recipe is on par with your friend who starts getting ready five hours before you go out. It's time consuming, and it requires a bit of concentration and a lot of patience. But, at the end of it, you'll have a gluten-free, low-lactose, FODMAP-friendly version of salted caramel shortbread (or caramel slice, or millionaire's shortbread, or whatever you want to call it). Good things come to those who spend hours making them.

Condensed milk

4 cups (1 L) lactose-free whole milk
1⅔ cups (370 g) superfine baker's or caster sugar

Shortbread

½ cup (50 g) almond meal
1 cup (120 g) tapioca flour
5 tablespoons (75 g) butter
2 tablespoons plus 2 teaspoons light brown sugar
1 egg

Caramel

7 tablespoons (100 g) butter
2 tablespoons light brown sugar
1½ teaspoons sea salt

Chocolate topping

7 ounces (200 g) dark chocolate, roughly chopped
1 teaspoon neutral oil (such as vegetable, canola, or grapeseed)

1. To make the condensed milk, combine the milk and superfine sugar in a large saucepan over medium heat and cook on a low boil, whisking intermittently, for 60 to 80 minutes. It should first turn a grey color before eventually thickening to a brown, condensed milk consistency. Be patient with it and keep watching. It might take longer than specified, or it might take less time—it depends on the milk and the stove.

2. To make the shortbread, preheat the oven to 350°F (180°C) and grease an 8-inch (20 cm) square baking pan.

3. Place all the ingredients in a food processor and process until everything is combined. It will be a sticky paste of a dough—transfer it to the fridge to firm up, if need be. Remove the dough from the processor and use your hands to gently press it until the mixture comes together. Scrape into the greased pan and, using swift movements or lightly oiled hands, use your palm to press the dough evenly into the pan.

4. Use a fork to prick a few holes in the shortbread, then bake in the oven for 10 minutes until lightly colored and slightly puffed up. Set aside to cool.

5. To make the caramel, melt the butter with the brown sugar in a small saucepan over medium heat. Whisk constantly, allowing the mixture to darken and begin bubbling, and then add the salt and condensed milk. Continue whisking for several minutes until thick and dark, then remove from the heat and cool slightly.

6. Pour the caramel over the cooled shortbread. Transfer to the fridge to chill and solidify completely.

7. To make the topping, melt the chocolate (using whichever method you like—I use a double boiler) and stir in the oil (this will help make it easier to slice later). Pour the chocolate over the caramel layer, working quickly but gently to spread the chocolate evenly before it starts to harden.

8. Refrigerate until the chocolate has solidified (about 1 or 2 hours) before slicing and serving.

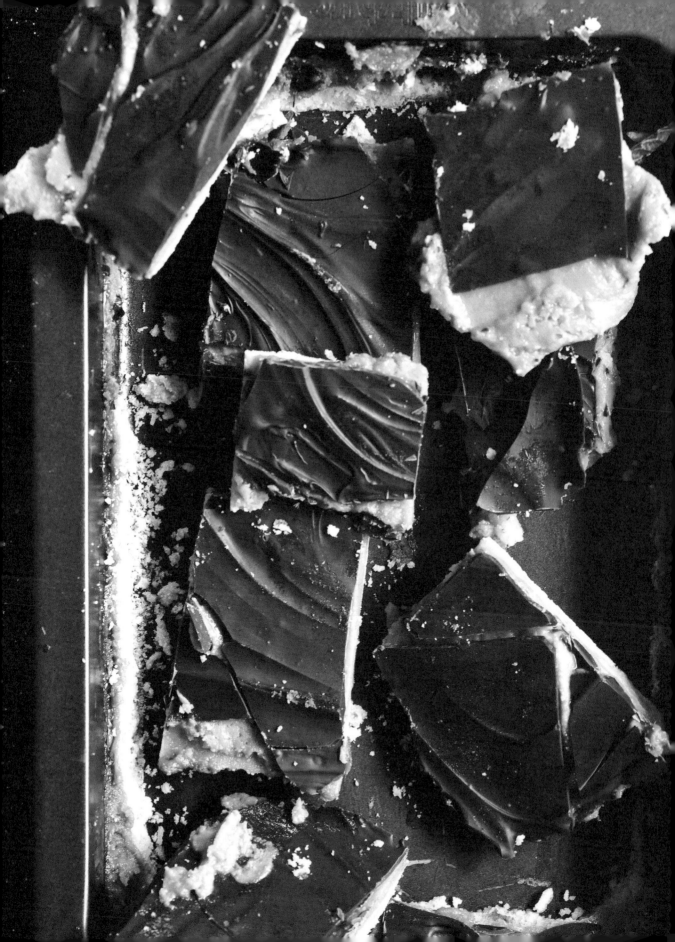

Strawberry Cobbler

SERVES
6 TO 8

Confession: My knowledge of cobbler has been derived exclusively from *Bon Appetit*'s YouTube channel. Controversial confession: I now like cobbler far more than I like pie. I've used summer strawberries for this cobbler, but you could use any low-fructose fruit you see fit. You could also use "regular people" fruit, if you're baking this for a gluten-free but otherwise "regular" person. You can serve this warm or cool, and with the remainder of the cream (ideally whipped with a tiny bit of confectioners' sugar) or vanilla ice cream (page 163).

Topping

1¼ cups (120 g) tapioca flour, plus extra for working the dough

¾ cup plus 3 tablespoons (120 g) white rice flour

¼ cup (55 g) superfine baker's or caster sugar

2 teaspoons baking powder

7 tablespoons (100 g) butter (salted or unsalted, but cold—straight from the fridge)

2 extra-large eggs, separately whisked well

½ cup plus 1 tablespoon (140 g) heavy cream (lactose-free is preferable)

Pinch of fine salt

Strawberries

2 pounds (1 kg) strawberries

2½ to 4 tablespoons superfine baker's or caster sugar

Pinch of sea salt flakes

Juice of 1 lemon

1 tablespoon orange blossom water (optional)

1 to 2 tablespoons gluten-free cornstarch (use less if using fresh and more if using frozen berries)

To finish

Crunchy sugar (such as turbinado)

1. **To make the topping,** combine the flours, superfine sugar, and baking powder.

2. Cut the butter into small cubes and add it to the flour mixture. Rub the butter pieces between your thumb and forefinger, so that they become little fine sheets of butter. Keep going until the mixture looks a little sandy. There should be no huge chunks of butter, but it shouldn't be entirely gone. If your butter starts melting, just pop the mixture in the fridge for 5 to 10 minutes.

3. Gently incorporate one whisked egg with a spoon. Add the cream, ¼ cup (60 g) at a time. Gently push the mixture around without flattening the pieces of butter. The dough should be shaggy, but all the loose bits of flour should be wet or attached to the main ball of dough. You might not need the last tablespoon of cream, but see how you go.

4. Gather the dough gently into a ball and flour a clean, dry surface with tapioca flour. Place the dough on the surface and gently create a rectangle of dough, a little over 1 inch (3 cm) thick. Keep moving the dough and making sure it isn't sticking. Add more flour, if necessary.

5. Preheat the oven to 400°F (200°C). Line a large baking sheet with parchment paper.

6. Use a biscuit cutter to cut out the cobbler bits, flouring it liberally and whenever necessary. Place the cut bits onto the lined baking sheet and continue until you have used all the dough. Depending on the size of your cutter, you should have 18 to 24 little topping bits. Place them in the freezer for a little while to set the butter.

7. **To prep the strawberries,** hull them and place in a large bowl. I like to leave some whole and chop the others for a bit of textural interest. Sprinkle the superfine sugar and salt into the bowl and massage it in. After a couple of minutes, add the lemon juice and orange blossom water, if using. Stir to combine, then add the cornstarch and stir.

8. Transfer the berries and all their juices to a 9 × 13-inch (23 × 33 cm) baking dish in an even layer. Remove the topping from the freezer and give each a brush of the remaining whisked egg. Arrange the pieces close together in the baking dish—a tight-knit pattern encourages them to expand upward in the oven, rather than outward.

9. Give the topping a sprinkle of crunchy sugar and place the dish in the oven. It's good practice to put a large baking sheet underneath, since fruit has a tendency to become juicy and run all over your oven floor. Bake for 10 minutes, then reduce the heat to 350°F (180°C) and bake for an additional 20 minutes. Remove from the oven, let cool, and serve.

Basic Vanilla Ice Cream

SERVES
6 TO 8

The rumors are true: Homemade ice cream is actually worth the effort and patience. This one is low-lactose by virtue of low-lactose dairy, but there is a low-FODMAP vegan variety on page 166. Once you master this basic ice cream, have a crack at mixing in new flavors—I like peanut butter and chocolate chip.

1¼ cups (300 g) whipping cream, (lactose-free is preferable)
1¼ cups (300 ml) lactose-free milk
¾ cup (165 g) superfine baker's or caster sugar
6 egg yolks
1 teaspoon vanilla bean paste or extract

1. In a medium saucepan over a medium-low heat, heat the cream, milk, and sugar together, mixing well to combine.

2. Whisk the egg yolks together in a bowl and set aside. Once the sugar and cream mixture is warm but not scalding, transfer a third of it into a pitcher and take the saucepan with the remaining mixture off the heat.

3. In a single, small stream, pour the pitcher of the hot cream mixture over the egg yolks, whisking constantly. This will heat the egg yolks without cooking or scrambling them. Once you have poured the entire pitcher into the eggs, return the saucepan to the heat. Pour the warmed egg yolk mixture into the pitcher and then pour that, in a thin stream, into the saucepan, whisking gently.

4. Continue to whisk the mixture gently over low heat until it coats the back of a spoon. Allow to cool, then transfer to a freezer-proof container. You can stir the ice cream mixture every couple of hours to discourage ice crystals from forming, or simply freeze until solid.

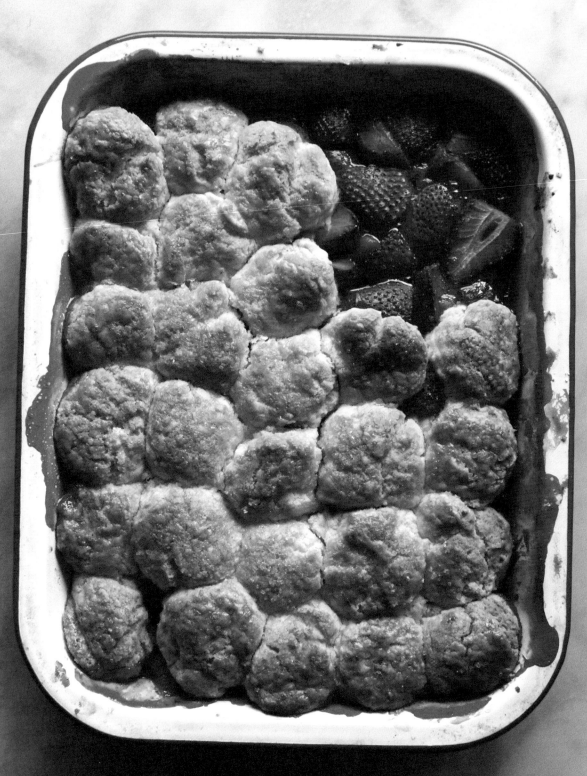

Strawberry Cobbler (page 162)

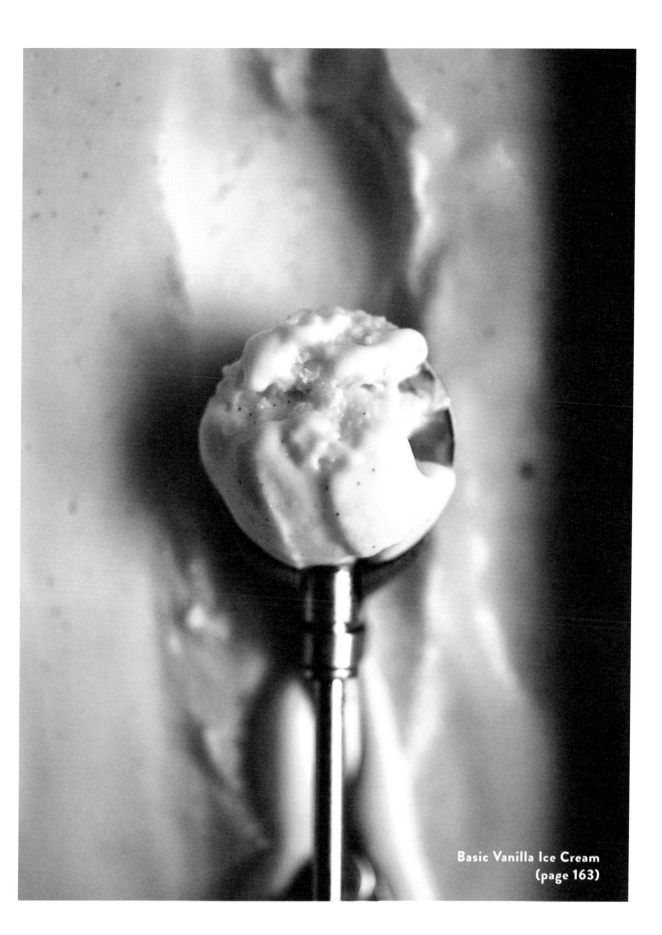

Basic Vanilla Ice Cream
(page 163)

Vegan Peanut Butter Ice Cream

SERVES
4 TO 6

All of the vegan ice cream recipes online seem to require one of the following: an ice-cream machine, a small fortune's worth of cashews or dates, or both, and a hell of a lot of bananas. In a (cashew) nutshell, not FODMAP-friendly, and not bench-space-friendly. This vegan ice cream isn't quite the traditional texture—the peanut butter gives it a bit of bite, but it is an excellent stand-in for the FODMAP-laden vegan variety.

Almond milk

1 cup (160 g) raw almonds

1 teaspoon vanilla bean paste or extract

Ice cream

1 cup (250 ml) coconut cream

⅔ cup (150 g) superfine baker's or caster sugar

¼ cup (65 g) natural peanut butter

1 teaspoon vanilla bean paste or extract

Pinch of sea salt

1. To make the almond milk, place the almonds in a large glass container along with the vanilla and 2½ cups (625 ml) water. Leave them to soak, covered and in the fridge, for at least 6 hours—overnight is ideal.

2. Transfer the nuts and their soaking water into a food processor or blender and blitz until smooth, roughly 2 minutes. Strain the milk using a nut milk bag, cheesecloth, or clean kitchen towel into a saucepan. You can discard the nut meal or use it to make the Cheesy Almond Crackers on page 196.

3. To make the ice cream, add the coconut cream and sugar to the saucepan and place over medium heat. Stir intermittently for 5 to 10 minutes, until the sugar has dissolved and the mixture starts to thicken slightly.

4. Add the peanut butter, vanilla, and salt and continue stirring intermittently for 5 to 10 minutes, until the mixture is smooth and slightly thickened. At that point, remove from the heat and let cool.

5. Transfer to a freezer-proof container. You can stir the mixture every couple of hours to prevent ice crystals from forming, or you can forget about it, leave it overnight, and come back when you're ready for some ice cream.

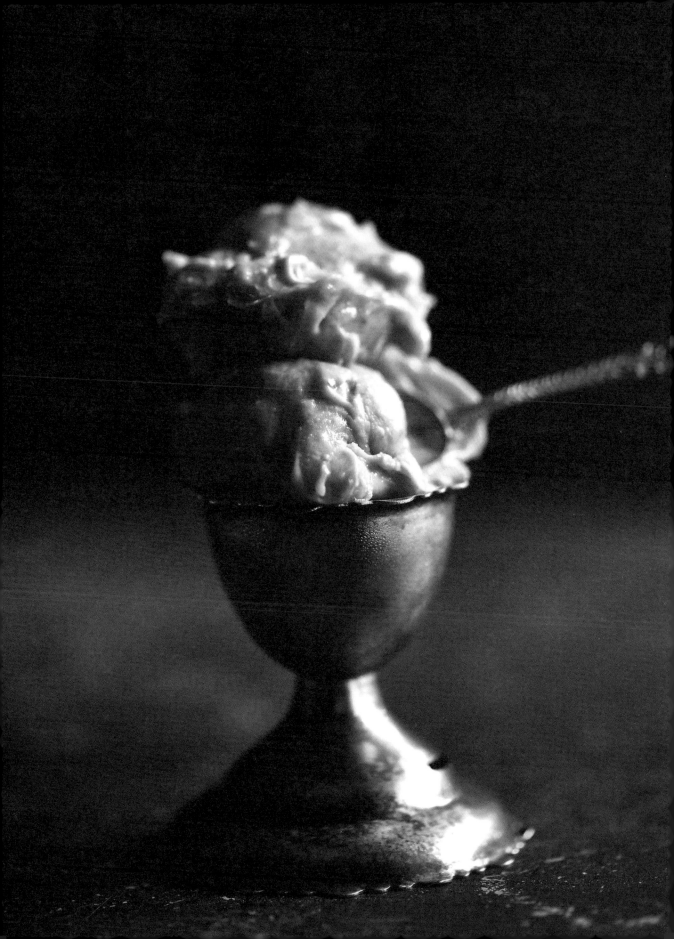

Pumpkin Pie

I know, I know. Homemade pumpkin purée! We don't have common access to canned pumpkin purée here in Australia, which is why my recipe uses the homemade variety. If you're a seasoned pumpkin pie expert, feel free to go rogue and use canned. While I'd love to include every tip I've written for this recipe, it is logistically impossible. You can find them all on my website if you're experiencing any recipe-related trepidation.

Pumpkin purée

1 small sugar pumpkin (you will use 1½ cups/300 g pumpkin purée)

Olive oil, for roasting

Pie crust

1 cup (130 g) fine white rice flour

¼ cup (25 g) tapioca flour, plus plenty extra for working the dough

¼ cup (25 g) glutinous rice flour

2 tablespoons plus 2 teaspoons superfine baker's or caster sugar

¼ teaspoon fine salt

6 tablespoons (90 g) good-quality butter, chopped into cubes and frozen for 10 to 15 minutes, plus extra for greasing

⅓ cup plus 1 tablespoon (100 g) lactose-free sour cream, frozen for 10 to 15 minutes

Ice water, only as needed

1 egg, whisked well

Filling

3 extra-large eggs

1 teaspoon ground cinnamon

1 teaspoon ground nutmeg

½ teaspoon ground clove

½ teaspoon ground ginger

¼ teaspoon fine salt

¾ cup (180 ml) maple syrup

¾ cup plus 2½ tablespoons (220 g) lactose-free cream or heavy cream

1. **To make the pumpkin purée,** preheat the oven to 325°F (160°C). Line a baking sheet with parchment paper. Cut the pumpkin into large chunks, remove the seeds, and brush with a light coating of oil. Roast in the oven on the lower rack for 40 minutes to an hour, until you can easily slice a knife through.

2. Remove from the oven and set aside to cool. Use your hands or a spoon to remove the pumpkin flesh from the skin, adding the flesh to a high-speed blender.

3. Purée the pumpkin until smooth. If your purée can be poured out of the processor easily, it contains too much liquid. To remove some liquid, pour the purée into a medium saucepan and cook over medium-low heat until it thickens. Set aside.

4. **To make the pie crust,** ensure that all your liquid ingredients are super cold. Put the butter and sour cream in the freezer, and put ice in your water.

5. Mix the flours, sugar, and salt together in a large mixing bowl. Add the cubes of cold butter and coat them with the flour mix. Use your fingertips to gently rub the butter into the flour mixture. Use your thumbs to push the butter up and back into the bowl. (I have a few YouTube tutorials on my website, if you're more of a visual learner.) The flour mixture should look a bit like damp sand.

6. Next, add the sour cream and mix gently with a spoon. Use your hands to gently bring the dough together without smushing the butter bits. If it comes together in a smooth-ish ball with no dry spots, don't add any water. If it is still dry and crumbly, add 1 teaspoon ice water. Use your hands to bring the dough together, then repeat with another teaspoon ice water, until the dough is smooth. Tightly wrap in a beeswax or plastic wrap and place in the fridge for 20 to 30 minutes.

recipe continues . . .

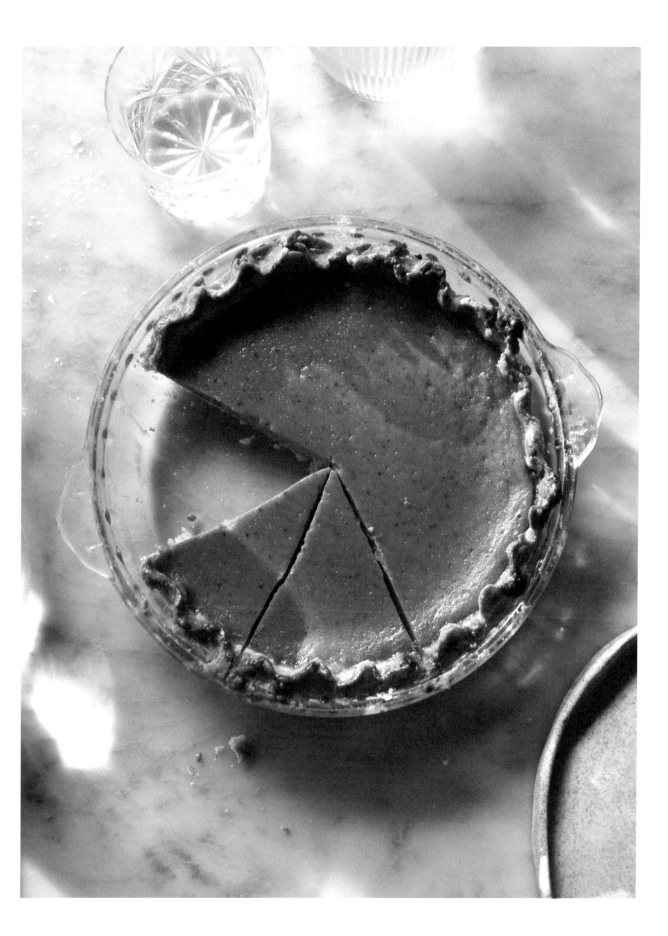

7. Generously grease a 10-inch (25 cm) deep-dish pie plate with butter and set aside. Liberally flour a piece of parchment paper a little larger than the pie plate with tapioca flour on a dry work surface. Place the dough in the center of the paper and flour it on the top, too. Use plenty of tapioca flour—it's the only way you'll come out with your sanity intact.

8. Gently roll the dough out, stopping every couple of rolls to flour both sides of the dough. "Turn" the dough regularly (pick it up and flip it over) to prevent it from sticking. Once the dough gets too big to turn, take another piece of well-floured parchment paper and place it on top. Working quickly, lift the dough up and flip it onto the newer piece of parchment paper. Then you can continue rolling. If, at any point, the dough becomes soft and difficult to work, place it flat in the fridge or freezer for a few minutes.

9. Once you have rolled it out to a couple of sizes larger than the pie plate, place it flat in the freezer for about 5 minutes. Gluten-free pastry is pretty sensitive, so be ready to patch up tears with your hands.

10. Lay the pastry flat on a working surface like a table so you have a bit of space underneath for your hands. Place the pie plate gently in the center of the pastry dough in whatever position maximizes pastry overhang.

11. Use one hand to pull a corner of the parchment paper toward you, and place the other directly underneath the center of the pie dish. As you pull the pastry off the table, the "catching" hand underneath will push the pastry into the pie dish, after which you will quickly flip the dish, letting the pastry fall into it. Don't stretch the pastry into the dish—be generous with letting it fall into the dish. Patch up any tears as necessary, then trim excessive overhang, redistributing it to places that may have none. Once the whole pie has equal overhang, fold it into the back of the pie dish to create a little wall of pastry. Do this the whole way around.

12. To crimp the pastry, use a knuckle of one hand to push the dough one way, and your thumb and pointer of the other hand to push into your knuckle, creating a crimp. Repeat the entire way around. Place the pie on a baking sheet so that you don't crush the crimps with fat oven mitt hands.

13. **To bake the pie crust,** preheat the oven to 350°F (180°C). Generously but gently brush the crimps of the pastry with the whisked egg.

14. Scrunch up a large piece of parchment paper, flatten it out again, and gently place it into the pastry. This will act as a guard between the pastry and your pie weights. Add the pie weights or dried beans, making sure they're pushing up against the walls of the crust.

15. Bake for 20 minutes. Gently lift out the paper and remove the pie weights. They will be very hot, so use the paper to transfer them to a heatproof dish to cool.

16. Place the crust back in the oven for 10 minutes, or until there are no raw bits of pastry on the bottom or edges.

17. Remove from the oven, brush the base, edges, and crimps with the egg wash, and bake for 1 to 2 minutes until set. Remove from the oven and set aside.

18. **To make the filling,** transfer the pumpkin purée to a large mixing bowl and crack in the eggs. Combine well, then add the spices and salt. Set aside.

19. Pour the maple syrup into a medium saucepan over medium heat. Once it starts bubbling, cook for 3 to 4 minutes. Add the cream in a couple of batches, stirring to combine before adding more. The mixture should look like a runny condensed milk. Remove from the heat.

20. Gently and slowly, so as not to curdle the eggs, stream the hot cream mixture into the pumpkin, stirring continuously. This will bring the eggs up to a warmer temperature and help create a silkier custard.

21. **To finish,** pour the filling into the pie crust. Bang the baking sheet gently a few times to remove any air—this will prevent bubbles on the top of your pie.

22. Bake for 30 minutes, or until the filling is mostly set but the center is still wobbly. Check regularly to ensure the filling hasn't gone crazy with cracks. (Cracks are a sign that there was too much liquid in the pumpkin or that the pie has been overcooked.)

23. As soon as the filling is cooked, turn the oven off. If you can, allow the pie to cool in the oven with the door held ajar by a wooden spoon. This will further ensure that cracks don't form.

24. Let the pie set before serving.

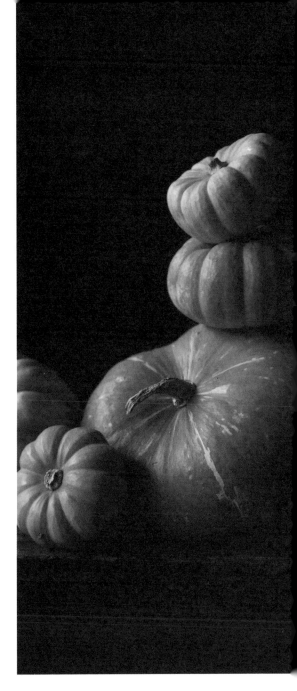

Easy Chocolate Cake with Brown-Butter Buttercream

MAKES ONE 8-INCH (20 CM) TWO-TIERED CAKE

My sister and I have a running joke where I gently mock her for a cake she used to make that was heavy on the oil. Truth is, the joke's on me: oil in cake is a revelation. This chocolate cake stays moist on the bench for as long as you have the willpower to leave it there.

Cake

1 cup (220 g) superfine baker's or caster sugar
½ cup (60 g) light brown sugar
1¼ cup (210 g) fine white rice flour
¾ cup (75 g) cocoa powder
2 teaspoons baking powder
1½ teaspoons baking soda
1¼ teaspoon fine salt
1 cup (240 ml) milk of choice
1 tablespoon apple cider vinegar
¾ cup (180 ml) vegetable oil
¼ cup (60 ml) freshly brewed espresso
2 teaspoons vanilla bean paste or vanilla extract
2 extra-large eggs
1 cup (235 ml) boiling water

Buttercream

½ cup plus 5 tablespoons (185 g) butter
1½ cups (180 g) confectioners' sugar
¾ cup (75g) cocoa powder
½ cup (120 ml) milk
½ teaspoon vanilla bean paste or vanilla extract (optional)
Pinch of fine salt

1. **To make the cake,** preheat the oven to 350°F (180°C). Grease and line the bottom of two 8-inch (20 cm) cake pans.
2. In a large bowl, combine the sugars, flours, cocoa powder, baking powder, baking soda, and salt, and whisk together until the mixture is a lovely chocolate brown.
3. In a small bowl, combine the milk and the vinegar and allow to sit for a few minutes to form a buttermilk. It might not curdle dramatically, but the buttermilk adds flavor and makes the cake fluffy.
4. In a medium bowl, combine the oil, espresso, vanilla, and eggs, then add to the dry ingredients. Whisk until a smooth batter has formed.
5. **To bloom the cocoa,** add the boiling water and whisk to combine. Pour into the pan and bake for 30 minutes, or until a skewer comes out clean. Remove and let cool.
6. **To make the buttercream,** place the butter in a small saucepan and brown very well over medium-low heat.
7. Pour the butter into a silicone cake mold and place in the freezer to set for about 20 minutes.
8. Break up the butter and put it in the bowl of a stand mixer with the whisk attachment. Beat until light and fluffy, scraping down the sides as necessary. Don't be fooled—this isn't a quick process. It will take about 15 minutes of beating and scraping down.
9. While the butter is mixing, sift the sugar and cocoa together. I hate sifting, so I wouldn't instruct you to do this unless it was totally necessary for a smooth frosting—I promise. Turn the speed to low and mix in with the milk, then add the salt and vanilla (stop the machine to add vanilla, or it gets tangled in the beaters).

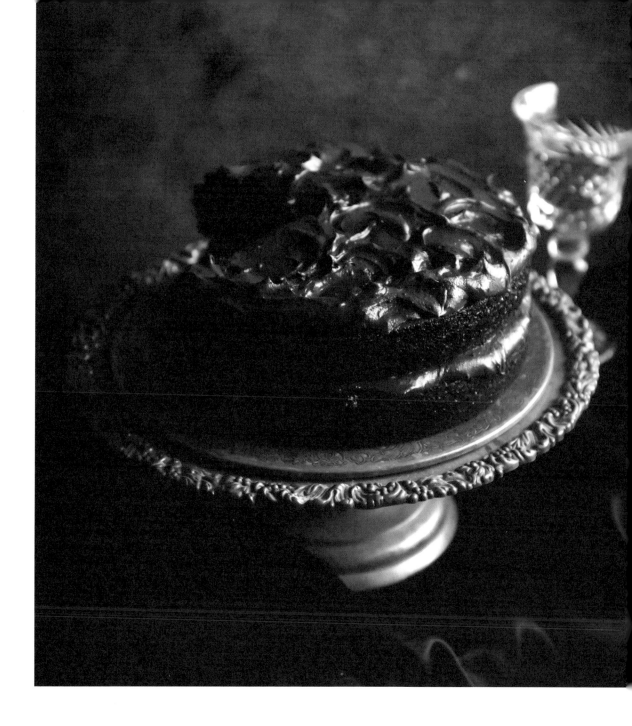

10. When the cakes are completely cool, it's time to assemble! Use an offset spatula or flat-edged knife to gently spread half the icing on top of each. Carefully place one on top of the other and then push down lightly to secure. Slice and serve. This keeps well in the fridge for a few days.

Salted Dark Chocolate Tart

SERVES
8 TO 10

An aesthetically pleasing, rich, silky smooth tart—a description not only of my aspirational future, but also of this gluten-free, grain-free, chocolate-centric delight. We're very lucky in Melbourne to have access to such a wide array of products catering to those of us with food intolerances, such as lactose-free cream, but I've included an option to substitute coconut cream for lactose-free cream, if you're unable to find it.

Tart crust

¾ cup (75 g) hazelnut meal
¾ cup (90 g) tapioca flour
½ cup (50 g) cacao powder
5 tablespoons (75 g) butter, roughly chopped
¼ cup (30 g) light brown sugar, not packed
1 egg

Chocolate filling

7 ounces (200 g) dark chocolate
1 cup (250 g) lactose-free cream or 1 cup (220 g) coconut cream
Good pinch of sea salt flakes, plus extra to serve
1 tablespoon freshly made espresso (optional)

1. **To make the tart crust,** preheat the oven to 350°F (180°C) and grease an 8-inch (20 cm) fluted tart pan.
2. Add all the ingredients for the crust to your food processor and blitz until you have a dough.
3. Gently press the dough into the pan and use a fork to prick little air holes in the bottom. Bake for 15 minutes.
4. **To make the filling,** while the tart base is baking, combine the chocolate and cream in a heatproof bowl. Place the bowl over a small saucepan of water over medium heat, making sure the bottom of the bowl doesn't touch the water. Allow the cream and chocolate to melt gently together until completely combined. Stir in the salt and espresso, if using. Remove from the heat.
5. **To finish,** once the crust has cooked, remove from the oven and cool slightly, then pour in the filling. Be careful not to touch the tart too much, or the top of the tart will have your grubby fingerprints on it!
6. Transfer to the fridge for at least 1 hour to set, sprinkle with some salt flakes, and serve.

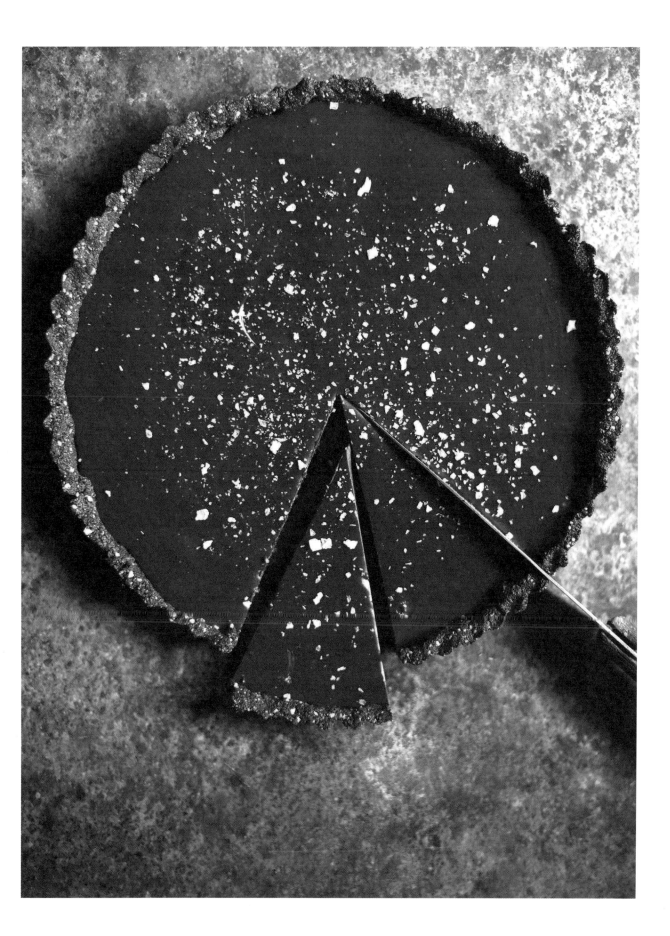

Lemon and Vanilla Cheesecake (on an Almond Crust)

MAKES ONE 8 X 4 INCH
(20 X 10 CM) LOAF
or 8 muffins

Revolutionary inventions: the internet, air travel, lactose-free cream cheese. Where it's regularly available, lactose-adverse folk can eat cheesecake with reckless abandon. I recommend using the full-fat variety of lactose-free cream cheese—you're worth it. Serve with a topping of your choosing (I like oven-roasted rhubarb and berries) and a light dusting of confectioners' sugar.

Almond crust

1 cup (100 g) almond meal

1 cup (120 g) tapioca flour

3 to 5 tablespoons (50–75 g) butter, diced

2 tablespoons plus 2 teaspoons light brown sugar

Cheesecake

26 ounces (750 g) lactose-free cream cheese, at room temperature

3 large eggs, at room temperature

½ cup (110 g) superfine baker's or caster sugar

⅓ cup (80 ml) freshly squeezed lemon juice (roughly 1 to 2 juicy lemons)

1 teaspoon vanilla bean paste or extract

1. **To make the crust,** preheat the oven to 350°F (180°C). Grease an 8-inch (20 cm) springform cake pan and line with parchment paper.
2. Combine all the ingredients in a food processor, starting with 3 tablespoons of the butter, and mix until a fine, moist crumb forms. It should come together if you compress a ball of it in your hand. If it doesn't, add a little more butter and mix again.
3. Using a firm hand, press the crumb into the prepared pan—it should be compact and even. Bake for 10 minutes, or until lightly golden. Set aside and allow to cool.
4. **To make the cheesecake,** beat the cream cheese and eggs with a stand mixer or in a large bowl until smooth. (Room temperature ingredients are super important to ensure the cheese component is smooth.) Add the sugar, lemon juice, and vanilla and continue to mix until the mixture is smooth.
5. Pour the cream cheese mixture into the crust. Bake for 30 to 40 minutes until the cheesecake is set but still bouncy.
6. Remove from the oven and run a knife around the edge (this will help avoid a big old crack down the middle) before allowing the cheesecake to cool.
7. Place in the fridge to chill for a couple of hours, or overnight, then slice and serve.

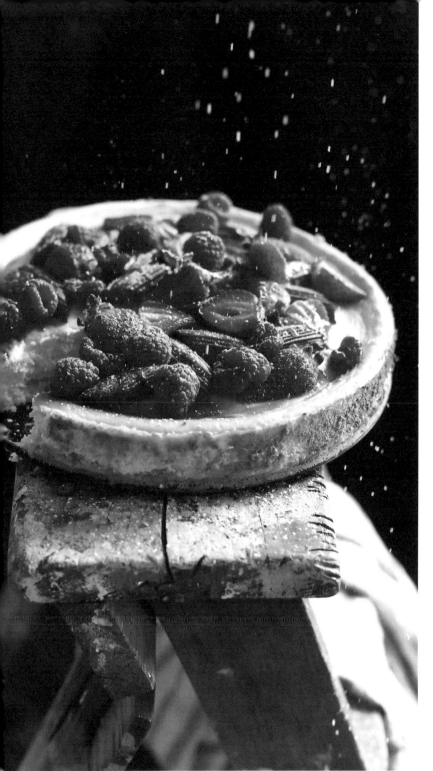
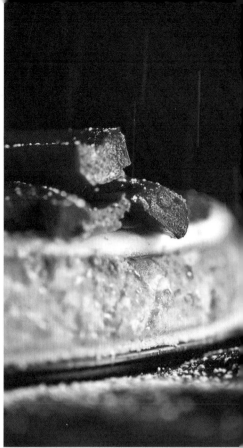

GETTING
SOCIAL

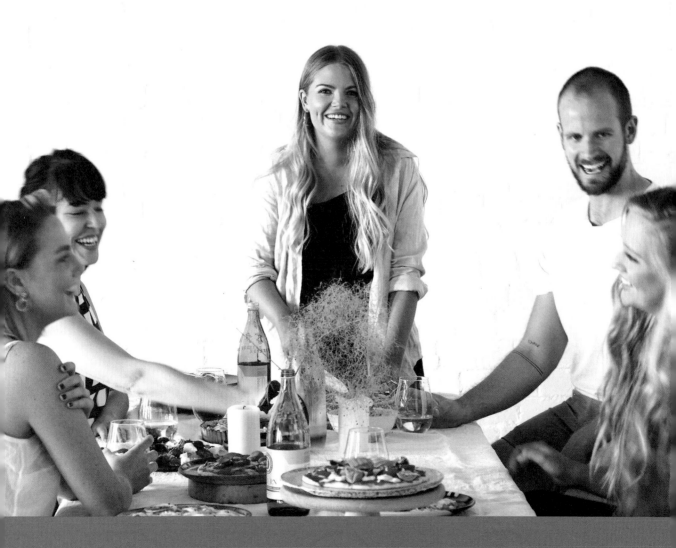

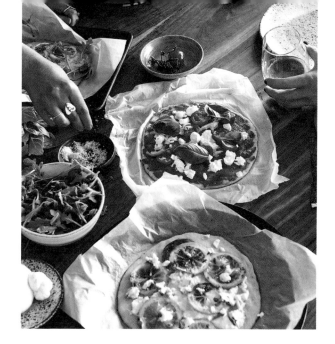

Although this chapter suggests a prerequisite social element to your evening, please don't feel obliged. As an extroverted introvert, I'm often compelled to host a Friday night pizza party, sans party or any people.

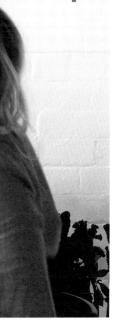

"Social" events, like any other day as an individual with digestive issues, can be fraught: people coming at you for a list of things you can eat, people blissfully ignoring your dietary restrictions, or (worst of all) people obliviously guzzling all your special options.

Solo or social, these recipes cover a whole host of occasions—from Christmas to a casual Saturday afternoon. My gift to you, introvert or extrovert—to make sure nobody eats all your special party snacks again. Is there anything more offensive than missing out on a minced pie come Christmas? Courtesy of a fruit-free fruit mince and a flaky gluten-free pastry, missing out is a thing of the past. This pastry can be used for pies and galettes all year round, too.

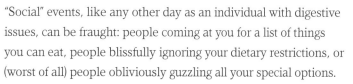

Mince Pies

I was today years old when I found out that mince pies aren't a common festive treat in the US like they are in Australia. Guys, you are missing out! Perfectly spiced fruit mince (or "fruit" mince, as the case may be) encased in a perfectly rich and crumbly pastry—what's not to love? This pastry can be used for pies and galettes all year round, too.

"Fruit" mince

3½ cups (500 g) diced kabocha squash, cut into roughly 5 mm cubes

1¼ cups (275 g) superfine baker's or caster sugar

⅓ cup plus 1½ tablespoons (100 ml) orange juice

⅓ cup plus 1½ tablespoons (100 ml) lemon juice

2½ tablespoons Campari

2 teaspoons ground cinnamon

2 teaspoons ground nutmeg

1 teaspoon ground clove

1 teaspoon vanilla bean paste or extract

2½ tablespoons cubed crystallized ginger (optional)

Sprig of rosemary (optional)

Pastry

1 cup (130 g) fine white rice flour

¼ cup (25 g) glutinous rice flour

¼ cup (25 g) tapioca flour

2 tablespoons plus 2 teaspoons superfine baker's or caster sugar

Pinch of fine salt

7 tablespoons (100 g) cold butter, cubed

⅓ cup plus 1 tablespoon (100 g) full-fat sour cream, chilled

2 teaspoons vanilla bean paste or extract

Chilled vodka or water, as needed

To finish

Butter, for greasing

2 teaspoons tapioca flour, plus extra for working the dough

1 egg, whisked well

Confectioners' sugar, for sprinkling (optional)

1. **To make the "fruit" mince,** combine all the ingredients and allow to sit in a nonreactive bowl overnight.

2. The next day (or at least 3 to 4 hours later), pour the mixture into a large saucepan or frying pan. Cook over medium-low heat and simmer for 30 minutes to an hour, stirring intermittently. The slower you cook the mixture, the softer the pumpkin will be, so if you have time, cook it low and slow. Eventually, a thickened syrup will form, while the squash pieces remain intact but soft. Remove from the heat and cool completely. If you have used the rosemary sprig, gently remove it and discard.

3. **To make the pastry,** combine the flours, sugar, and salt in a large mixing bowl, stirring to combine. Rub in the butter, using your forefinger and thumb to press the butter and flour together. The end result should be the consistency of damp sand, with small but visible pieces of butter throughout the mixture.

4. Add the cold sour cream and vanilla and use a spoon to stir until mostly incorporated. Use your hands to bring the dough together into a ball that is smooth and easy to handle—not too craggy and dry, but also not too wet that it sticks to your hands. To that end, add vodka by the teaspoon and only as necessary— even if it's just a teaspoon to bring it all together. Wrap in beeswax or plastic wrap and refrigerate for around 30 minutes.

5. **To make the mince pies,** preheat the oven to 350°F (180°C) and grease a 12-cup muffin pan liberally with butter.

recipe continues . . .

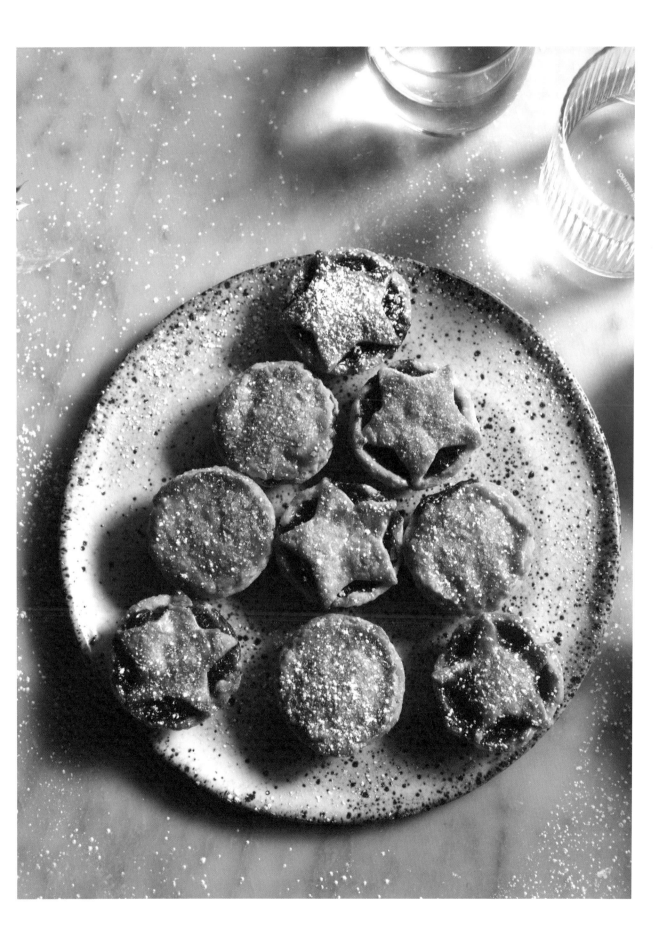

6. Liberally (tapioca) flour a large piece of parchment paper on a dry, clean bench. Place the dough on the sheet and liberally flour the top. Cut off about a quarter of the pastry to set aside for the tops of the pies. Roll the remaining pastry out into a large, rough rectangle, about 5 mm thick. If the pastry cracks, allow it to warm up a little. If it's too soft to handle, pop it in the fridge for 5 minutes.

7. Use a circular cutter significantly larger than the muffin cups to cut out 12 bottom crusts. Lower each pastry round into a muffin pan cup, gently pressing it flush against the sides without stretching the dough. Any tears can easily be patched up with your fingers, and excessive dough around the edges can be neatly trimmed. Set aside.

8. Stir the 2 teaspoons tapioca flour into the mince until it's well combined.

9. Fill the pastry with the mince and refrigerate while you make the top crusts.

10. Roll the reserved pastry out into a 5 mm thick rectangle, flouring liberally whenever necessary. Use a cutter the same size or a little bigger than the muffin pan cups to cut out 12 circles and/or stars for top crusts.

11. Preheat the oven to 350°F (180°C) and remove the filled crusts from the fridge. Use the egg to lightly egg-wash the sides of the pies, then press the top crusts gently but firmly atop to secure. Paint the tops with egg wash and sprinkle with confectioners' sugar, if using.

12. Bake for 20 minutes, or until they smell fragrant and have colored lightly. Turn the broiler on and continue to bake for another couple of minutes, watching closely. Remove when they are golden brown on top.

13. Serve the pies warm or cold. Store in an airtight container for up to a week.

Brie Cranberry Wreath with Flaky Pastry

SERVES 8 TO 12

I obviously spend too much time on the internet looking at American bloggers' culinary pursuits; my Australian friends were decidedly wary when I introduced a "brie and cranberry wreath" to Friendmas. I won them over with it, though, so the world can go on. We don't have access to many fresh cranberries here, so I used frozen. Whatever you do, don't used dried—they're much higher on the FODMAP front.

Pastry

7 tablespoons (100 g) cold butter, diced
⅓ cup plus 1 tablespoon (100 g) full-fat sour cream
Ice water, only as needed
1 cup (130 g) fine white rice flour
¼ cup (25 g) tapioca flour, plus extra for working the dough
¼ cup (25 g) glutinous rice flour
½ teaspoon fine salt

Filling

1½ cups (150 g) fresh or frozen cranberries, but not dried
¼ cup (55 g) superfine baker's or caster sugar
Pinch of ground clove
Grating of fresh nutmeg

To finish

1 wheel of brie, camembert, or a lactose-free alternative, thinly sliced and each slice cut into thirds
1 egg, whisked well

1. **To make the pastry,** ensure that all your liquid ingredients are super cold. Put the butter and sour cream in the freezer, and put ice in some water.
2. Mix the flours and salt together in a large mixing bowl. Add the butter and coat with the flour mix. Use your fingertips to gently rub the butter into the flour mixture. (I have a few YouTube tutorials on my website if you're more of a visual learner.) It should look a bit like damp sand.
3. Use a spoon to gently incorporate the sour cream. Use your hands to gently bring the dough together without smushing the butter bits too much.
4. If your dough comes together in a smooth-ish ball with no dry spots, don't add any water. If it is still dry and crumbly, add 1 teaspoon ice water. Use your hands to bring the dough together, then repeat with another teaspoon until the dough is smooth.
5. Tightly wrap the dough in beeswax or plastic wrap and refrigerate for 20 to 30 minutes.
6. **To make the filling,** combine all the ingredients with 1 tablespoon water in a small saucepan over medium-low heat. Cook for 10 minutes, until the cranberries are thawed (if using frozen) and the liquid has become more of a cranberry syrup. Set aside to cool.
7. **To finish,** preheat the oven to 400°F (200°C). Once the cranberries have cooled, liberally dust a large sheet of parchment paper with tapioca flour on a large, dry surface.
8. Bring your pastry to a temperature at which you can roll it out. You can tell if it's ready to roll (lol) because it will be a little flexible and malleable under the weight of the rolling pin. If it's hard and cracks when you try to roll it, give it a little extra time on the bench.

recipe continues . . .

9. When it's ready, gently give the dough a few whacks with the rolling pin to encourage it into a rough circle shape. From there, gently roll out the pastry into a large circle (size doesn't matter too much, as long as the pastry is roughly 5 mm thick), moving it around every few rolls to ensure it hasn't stuck to the parchment paper. Use as much tapioca flour as necessary. If the dough gets too warm, pop it back into the fridge. If the butter pieces melt, the pastry will lose its puff.

10. Flour the top of the dough liberally. Take another piece of parchment paper and use a gentle but quick motion to flip the pastry over onto the new parchment sheet. I use one hand to pull the parchment paper to the edge of the table and the other to place under the pastry and flip it over. This is to ensure that the pastry isn't stuck to the original parchment sheet while cooking.

11. Take a small-medium circular bowl (this will be the center of the wreath) and lightly imprint it in the center of the dough. *Do not* press it down to cut a hole, just enough to form a circle imprint. Use a sharp, non-serrated knife to cut four equally spaced lines through the center of just this inner circle, as if slicing a pizza and forming eight even triangular "slices," but with the outer edges still attached to the rest of the dough circle. (Have a look at the YouTube video linked on my website, because it's a simple process but hard to describe.) These pieces will pull up and out over the pastry to form the wreath.

12. Paint the cranberry mixture evenly around the center star, leaving some space on the outer edges to pull them up over the filling. Top with the brie.

13. Gently pull up the outer edges of the pastry and press them into the filling to secure them. They should reach about halfway across the filling.

14. Gently flip up one little triangle of the inner star and fold it up over the filling, adjoining the outer edges of pastry and creating the little inner star. Repeat with the remaining triangles, ensuring they have adhered to the outer pastry (or else the wreath will become a volcanic mess of brie in the middle).

15. Brush with the egg. Gently slide the wreath onto a baking sheet (this is easiest by gently but quickly pulling it off the table and onto the baking sheet) and bake for 20 minutes.

16. Give the wreath an extra brush with the egg wash to patch up any cracks. Return to the oven for another 10 or so minutes, until the top is golden brown and the brie is bubbling. This is best served straight from the oven but is delicious when cooled, too.

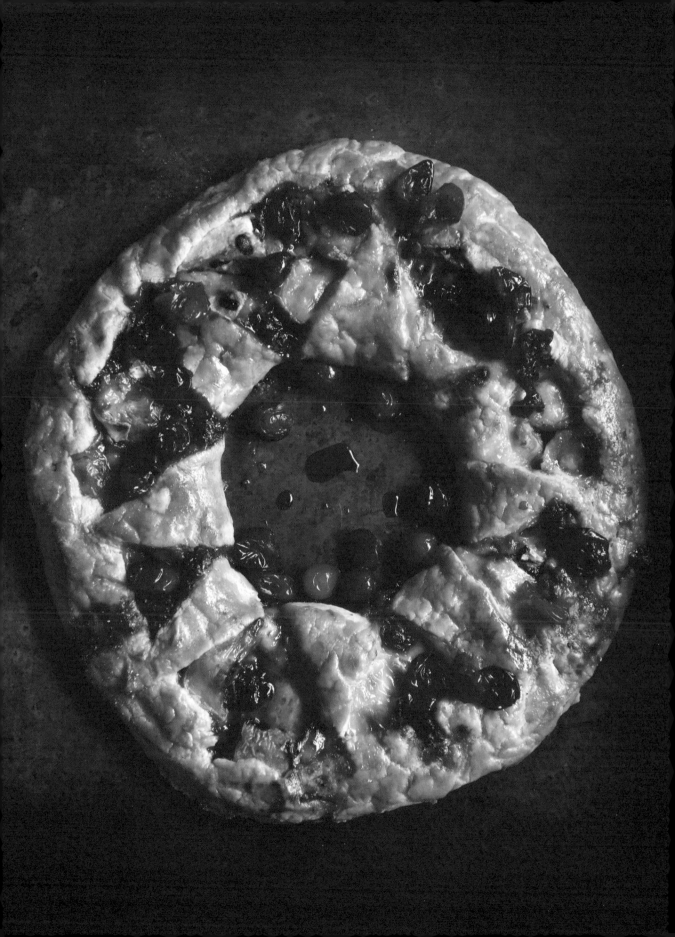

From-Scratch Bloody Mary

SERVES 4

Although I'm fully aware of the miraculous restorative qualities of a Bloody Mary on a Sunday afternoon, I am one of the rare breed that enjoys the drink whether I've had a night on the tiles or a night in bed. I had a revelatory Bloody Mary experience at a South American–inspired restaurant in Hobart, Tasmania, where they used a homemade roasted vegetable mix as the base of the drink. I've tried to emulate that to the best of my ability here, roasting the peppers for sweetness and a little twist. Labor intensive, yes—but worth it for the Bloody Mary enthusiasts among us, not to mention a surefire way to avoid sneaky fructose in store-bought juice.

2 red bell peppers
5 tomatoes (roughly 2 pounds/
    1 kg)
Olive oil spray
½ cup (125 ml) vodka
¼ cup (60 ml) apple cider
    vinegar
2½ tablespoons light brown
    sugar
1 tablespoon gluten-free tamari
1 teaspoon horseradish cream
¼ teaspoon smoked paprika
¼ teaspoon ground cinnamon
Good dash of Tabasco

To finish (all optional)
Ice, for serving
2 celery ribs, halved crosswise
Cucumber slices or lemon
    wedges
Green Sicilian (Castelvetrano)
    olives

1. Preheat the oven to 350°F (180°C). Place the peppers and tomatoes on separate baking sheets and spray lightly with oil. Roast the tomatoes for around 20 minutes, until they are browned and blistered, and roast the peppers for an additional 10 to 20 minutes, depending on their size, until they are soft and blistered. Place them in a bowl, cover with a plate or kitchen towel to encourage sweating, and leave to cool.

2. Once the vegetables are cool enough to handle, peel the peppers and remove and discard the stems and seeds.

3. Transfer the vegetables to a food processor along with all the other ingredients and 1½ cups (375 ml) water, whizzing and adjusting for taste as you see fit. Pour straight into serving glasses. If you absolutely hate "bits" in your drink, you can strain the juice through a loose-holed sieve. Keep in mind that a) you'll be there a long time, b) you'll lose a considerable amount of drink, and c) surely the fiber from the veggies will assist your hangover.

4. Add ice, if you like, then serve with half a celery rib, cucumber slices or lemon wedges, and plenty of olives.

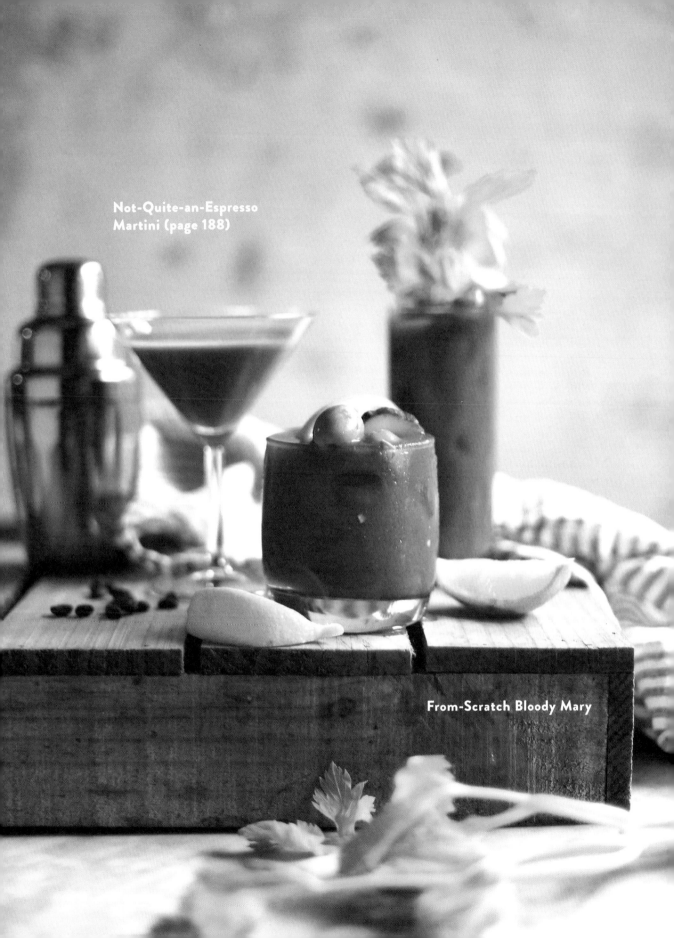

Not-Quite-an-Espresso
Martini (page 188)

From-Scratch Bloody Mary

Not-Quite-an-Espresso Martini

SERVES 1

Blasphemous. Potentially regrettable. Very basic. Those are a few words to describe the inclusion of my homemade pre-drink-style martini in a book. That said, if you're anything like me, you'll be thrilled to know that it's possible to whip up a few "espresso martinis" at home, with naught but everyday fridge items.

2 tablespoons (30 ml) vodka
2 tablespoons (30 ml) freshly made espresso
1 tablespoon plain coconut yogurt
1 teaspoon maple syrup
Dash of vanilla bean paste or extract
Ice, for serving

1. Place all of the ingredients in a blender and process until smooth.
2. Serve in chilled glasses, over ice.

Pizza Crusts

MAKES
3 OR 4
CRUSTS

Psyllium husk strikes again, this time holding together the easiest, crunchiest gluten-free pizza crusts that—wait for it—have bottoms that are crispy instead of soggy. There are two choices for flours, which work equally well: Brown rice flour gives a more traditional appearance, while tapioca flour creates a chewier crust. Both delicious.

1 cup (250 ml) warm water
One ¼-ounce (7 g) packet active dry yeast
2 teaspoons white sugar
2 tablespoons psyllium husk
½ cup (120 ml) olive oil, plus extra to grease your hands
⅔ cup (160 ml) boiling water
1 cup (160 g) potato starch
1 cup (130 g) fine white rice flour (make sure it's finely ground or the texture will be grainy)
¼ cup (30 g) tapioca or fine brown rice flour
1 to 2 teaspoons fine salt

1. Mix together the warm water, yeast, and sugar and set aside for 10 to 15 minutes to activate. Discard and begin again if the mixture hasn't bubbled after that time.
2. Whisk the psyllium husk and oil together in a mixing bowl until it begins to thicken a little, then add the boiling water. Whisk for a couple of minutes until it comes together in a thick, slimy blob. (Appetizing, I know.) Set aside.
3. Combine the potato starch, flours, and salt in a large bowl. Add the bubbly yeast mixture and the psyllium husk blob. Using your hands, mix until completely combined (squelch the dough through your fingers—you'll see what I mean—to incorporate everything evenly).
4. Cover the bowl with a kitchen towel and place in a warm, draft-free place for 1 hour, or until it rises by about half. In winter, atop a heating vent or an oven in use is ideal. In summer, a nice sunny spot indoors is perfect.
5. Preheat the oven to 350°F (180°C) and line four round pizza pans with parchment paper.
6. Use a teaspoon or so oil to grease your hands and then divide the dough into four balls. Gently press the dough into rounds on each of the lined pans (if you'd like a thick crust, see the Note). Leave to rest for 5 minutes, then bake for 5 to 10 minutes. After this, you're ready to start topping them (see next page for ideas and cooking instructions).

Note: For a thick crust, use a fork to flip the edges of the dough toward the center of the pizza. Then, using the parchment paper, gently flip the pizza over onto a new sheet of parchment paper. The crimps will now be underneath, forming a thick crust.

recipe continues . . .

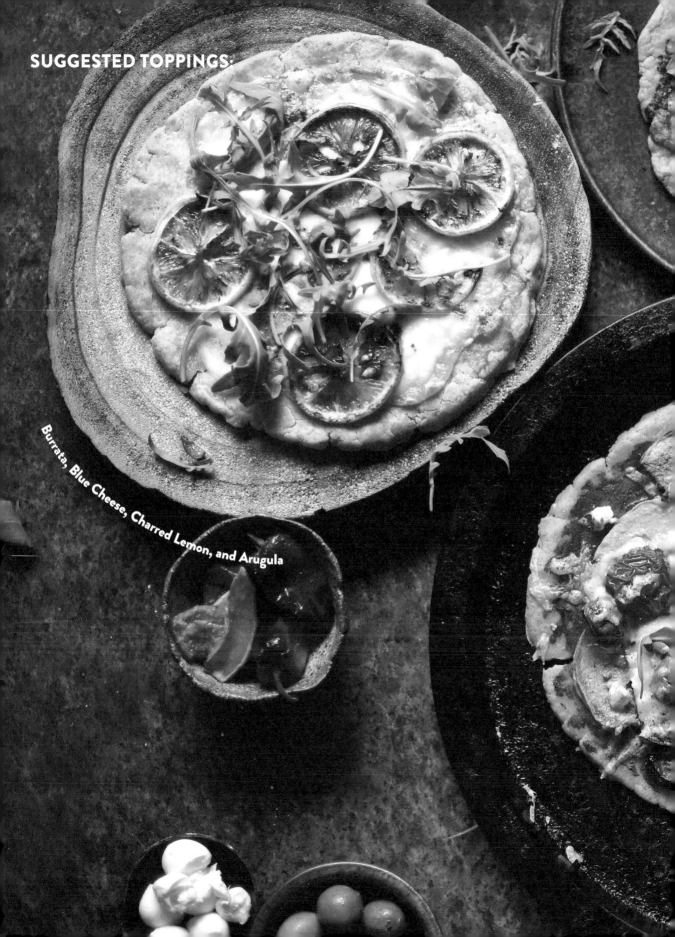

SUGGESTED TOPPINGS:

Burrata, Blue Cheese, Charred Lemon, and Arugula

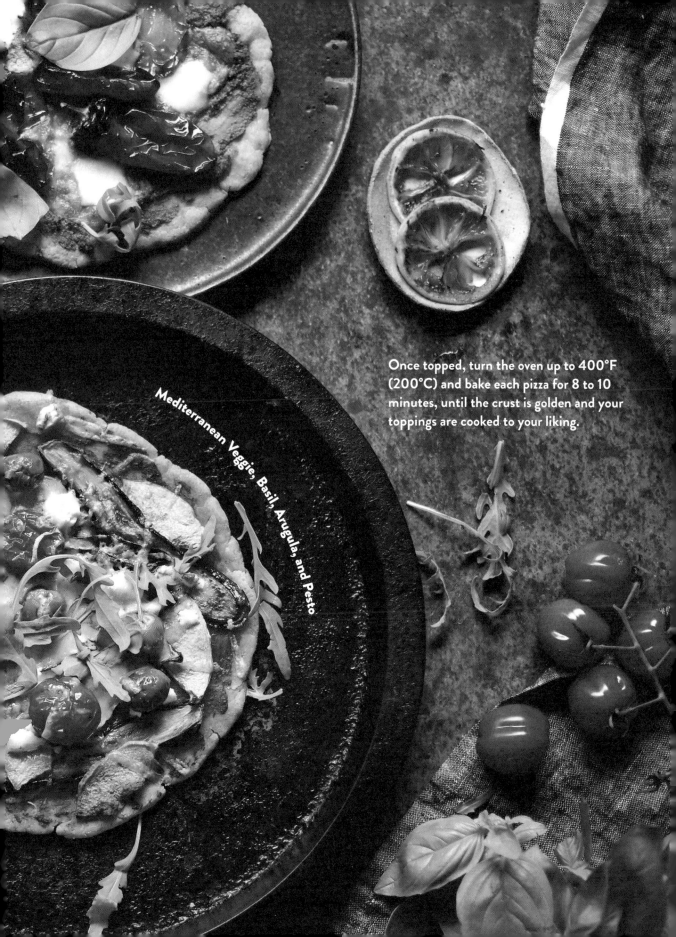

Mediterranean Veggie, Basil, Arugula, and Pesto

Once topped, turn the oven up to 400°F (200°C) and bake each pizza for 8 to 10 minutes, until the crust is golden and your toppings are cooked to your liking.

Piña Coladas

SERVES 4

Piña Coladas

Rupert needn't have asked the question—everyone likes piña coladas. Even low-FODMAPpers, because pineapple gets the tick of approval in servings up to half a cup.

2 cups (350 g) fresh pineapple chunks
Juice of 1 lime
1 tablespoon light brown sugar
½ cup (120 ml) coconut milk
½ cup (120 ml) coconut water
¼ cup (60 ml) rum
Ice, for serving

Blend the pineapple until smooth, then strain to get rid of any stringy bits. Add the remaining ingredients and blend. Serve with ice.

Passion Fruit Caipirinha

Passion Fruit Caipirinha

There's not a lot in life I can say I'm an expert at, but spending all my money on expensive cocktails is one activity in which I have undoubtedly achieved my 10,000 hours. While working a photography job for a restaurant group in Melbourne, my friend/ hand model and I started making a routine pit stop at our favorite cocktail bar after all our "hard work." I quickly became enamored with caipirinhas—a Brazilian mojito, made with a Brazilian liquor called cachaça. For the everyday person who actually values having life savings, you can substitute cachaça with a dark rum, making this drink a passion fruit mojito. I've used coconut sugar here to "healthify" this cocktail as much as one can, but you can also use light brown sugar, and more of it than this if you've got a particularly sweet tooth.

2½ tablespoons cachaça
2 teaspoons coconut sugar
1 lime, cut in wedges
Ice, to fill the glass
Pulp of ½ a large passion fruit

1. Combine the liquor, sugar, and ¼ cup (60 ml) water in a cold glass and stir until the sugar has dissolved.
2. Run a slice of lime around the edge of a glass and then fill with ice and a few lime wedges. Pour the liquor over the ice and finish with the passion fruit pulp. Stir and serve.

Salted Honey and Sage Baked Camembert with a Baklava Crumb

SERVES 4 TO 6
(depending on the
size of camembert)

I don't have a religion, but if I did, its main tenet would be that it's not a party until some form of baked cheese appears. While honey is high in fructose, the quantity you'll consume if you plan to share this dish (this is a no-judgment zone, by the way) shouldn't be an issue. A whole baked camembert to yourself, on the other hand . . .

Baked cheese

One 8- to 9-ounce (about
250 g) wheel good-quality
Camembert
About 10 small sage leaves
1 teaspoon honey, warmed
(you can substitute with
maple syrup, if you're hyper-
intolerant)
Sprinkle of sea salt

Baklava crumb

½ cup (50 g) walnuts
2 teaspoons honey
1 teaspoon ground cinnamon
Pinch of ground nutmeg

To serve (optional)

Cheesy Almond Crackers
(page 196)
1 bunch red grapes, roasted
for 20 to 30 minutes at 350°F
(180°C)

1. **To bake the cheese,** preheat the oven to 350°F (180°C). Gently score the Camembert across the top and very carefully fold and stuff the sage leaves into the scores.

2. Place the Camembert in an ovenproof dish, or back in the box it came in (provided it is wooden, as pictured), and place it on a baking sheet. Drizzle the honey over the Camembert and finish with the salt. Place in the oven for 5 minutes.

3. **Meanwhile, to make the baklava crumb,** combine all the ingredients in a food processor and whizz until a sticky crumb has formed. Place three quarters of this crumb atop the Camembert and return to the oven for 5 to 10 minutes. Keep an eye on it and remove it as soon as it begins to look and feel like a waterbed—any longer and it will harden.

4. **To serve,** transfer to a serving plate and top with the remaining baklava crumb. Serve with Cheesy Almond Crackers and roasted red grapes, if you like.

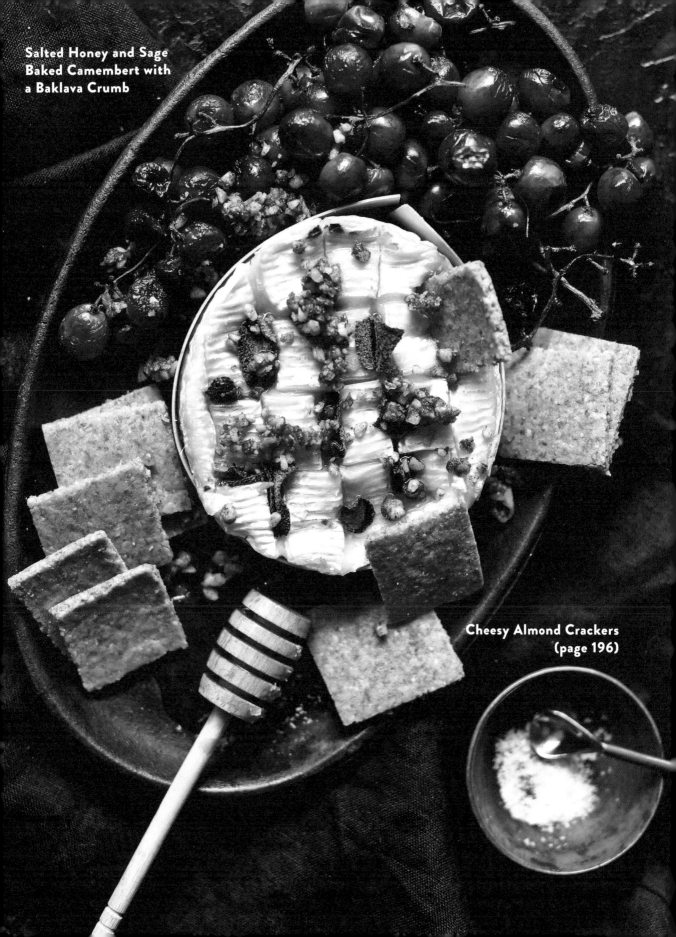

Salted Honey and Sage Baked Camembert with a Baklava Crumb

Cheesy Almond Crackers (page 196)

Cheesy Almond Crackers

MAKES 15 TO 20 CRACKERS

These crackers were inspired by a cheesy variety of gluten-free crackers that I discovered at the mecca that is Whole Foods while I was in New York.

½ cup (70 g) sunflower seeds
1 cup (100 g) almond meal
1 tablespoon psyllium husk
½ cup (50 g) grated vegetarian
  Parmesan
1 teaspoon smoked paprika
1 tablespoon olive oil
1 teaspoon fine salt

1. Preheat the oven to 350°F (180°C). Tear off two big sheets of parchment paper and get a baking sheet ready.
2. Blitz the sunflower seeds in a food processor until they are fine and meal-like. Add the remaining ingredients along with 2½ tablespoons water and process just until the dough comes together.
3. Sandwich the dough between the two sheets of parchment paper and gently roll out into a thin, even sheet. Remove the top sheet of parchment paper and transfer the bottom sheet with the rolled dough onto the baking sheet. If you're working in particularly warm conditions, you can put the mixture in the fridge for 30 minutes to solidify.
4. Bake for 10 to 12 minutes, until the crackers are golden but not burnt. Cut into pieces immediately and allow to cool before serving—they firm up as they cool. For particularly crunchy crackers, return the sliced crackers to the oven for an additional 3 to 5 minutes. Store any leftovers in an airtight container and eat within the week, if they last that long.

Vegan Chocolate Irish Cream

SERVES 4

I was rather naive as to the caloric value of Irish cream until I made a lactose-free version myself. I'm not one to shy away from a calorie, but a line must be drawn somewhere, and this is mine. By making the almond "cream" (which is a thicker almond milk) yourself, you have full control over not only the thickness, but also the additives and preservatives, or lack thereof. A nut milk bag is easy to buy online, or from a health food store. If vegan Irish cream won't convince you of the merits of homemade nut milks, I'm afraid you're a lost cause. (Not really, but you should definitely make your own nut milk.)

Almond "cream"

2 cups (320 g) raw almonds
1 teaspoon vanilla bean paste or extract
Pinch of sea salt

Irish cream

½ cup (60 g) light brown sugar, not packed
½ cup (125 ml) Irish whisky or rum
2½ tablespoons freshly made espresso
2 ounces (50 g) vegan chocolate, melted
Ice, to serve

1. **To make the almond "cream,"** place the almonds in a large glass jar and cover with 4 cups (1 L) water. Add the vanilla and salt, then soak for at least 6 hours—overnight is best.
2. Transfer the almonds and their soaking water to a blender and blitz for 2 minutes. Using a nut milk bag, cheesecloth, or clean, dry kitchen towel, strain the milk into a container. You can discard the nut meal, but I like to use it to make crackers—there are loads of recipes online, or you can use 1 cup for the Cheesy Almond Crackers on page 196.
3. **To make the Irish cream,** transfer 1½ cups (375 ml) of the almond "cream" to a saucepan with the sugar. Cook for 10 to 15 minutes, until the mixture has thickened and has a consistency somewhat similar to condensed milk.
4. Transfer to the blender along with the whisky, espresso, and the remaining almond "cream" and blitz to combine. While the motor is running, pour in the chocolate in a thin stream. Add ice to four glasses, pour in the Irish cream, and serve.

Mulled Wine

What a festive, warming and wintry delight mulled wine is. Unless, of course, you're sitting in 100°F/40°C heat on Christmas Day wondering why you didn't wear a more breathable shirt, as we do in Australia. With that in mind, I've taken one for the team by extensively testing the concept of iced mulled wine, which I can assure you from experience will quell your sweat mustache while also delivering that festive feel. I've also added an unrefined sugar, though to a lesser degree than a standard mulled wine, because I always find mulled wine unbearably sweet. Given the quantities I drink it in, I'd rather just have a headache from the wine and skip the sugar hangover.

One 750 ml bottle merlot or other red wine
⅓ cup (65 g) coconut sugar
2 cinnamon sticks
3 star anise
1 teaspoon vanilla bean paste or extract
4 black peppercorns
Good pinch of ground nutmeg
Ice (optional)

1. Combine all of the ingredients (except the ice, of course) in a large pot and place over low heat for 10 to 15 minutes, until fragrant. Ensure the wine doesn't come to a boil, or the alcohol content will evaporate—a real tragedy!
2. Serve warm, or allow to cool and serve over ice, if desired.

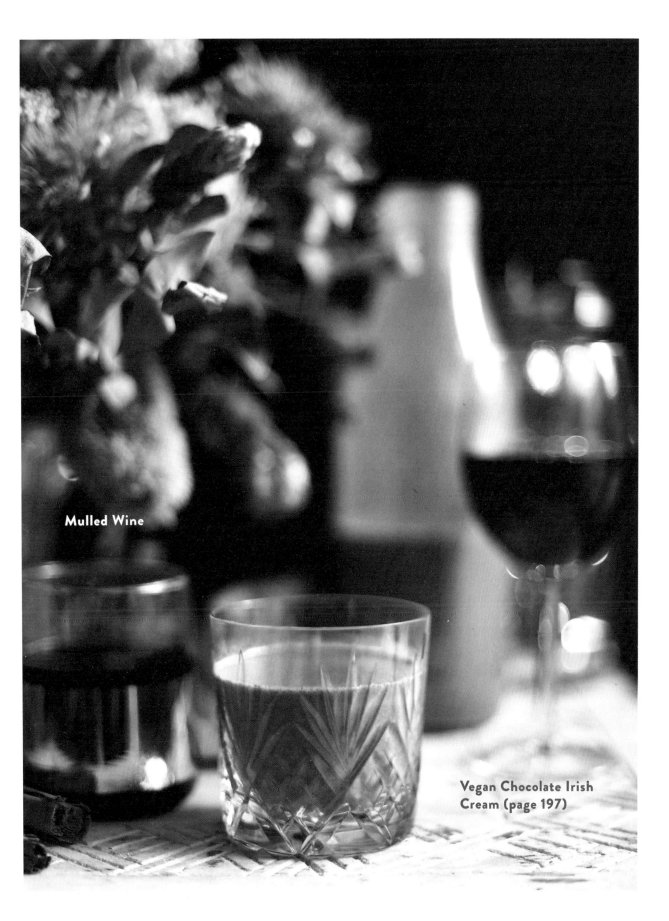

Mulled Wine

Vegan Chocolate Irish
Cream (page 197)

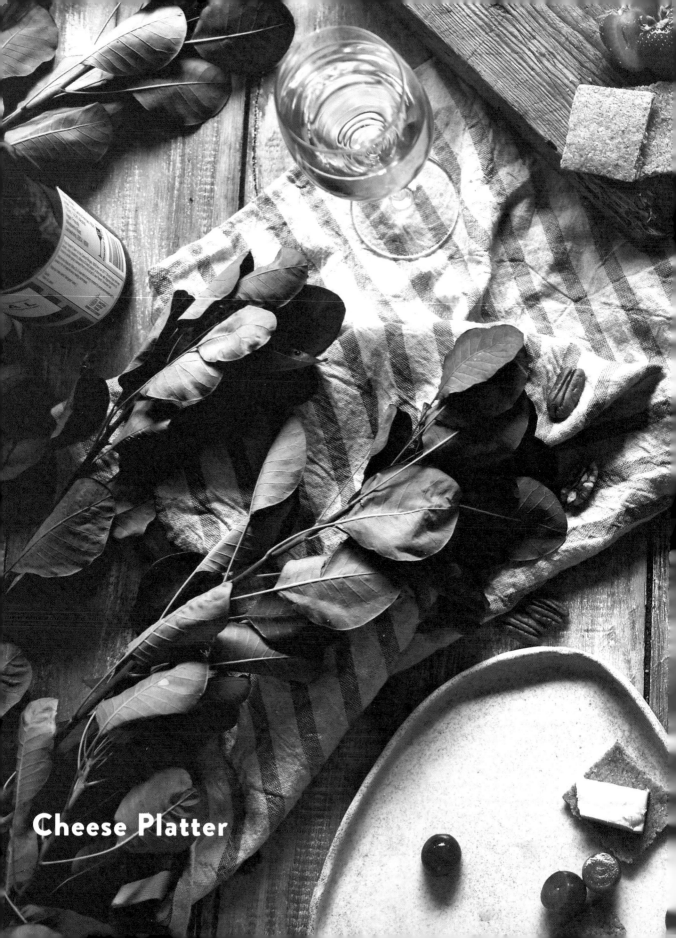

Cheese Platter

Pint of fresh strawberries

A bunch of grapes, red or green

A ripe blue cheese (such as Stilton)

Firm ripened cheese (such as Parmesan, pecorino, Swiss, or cheddar)

Camembert

Brie or a log of goat cheese

A batch of Cheesy Almond Crackers (page 196)

2 handfuls of FODMAP-friendly nuts and/or seeds, like pine nuts, walnuts, or sunflower seeds

2 ounces (50 g) dark chocolate, roughly chopped

Red Pepper and Feta Dip

Given the number of dips available at the supermarket, I naively assumed they'd be tedious to make at home. Not so! A blender, an oven, and an enthralling episode of *Law and Order: SVU* are all you need to pass the time while you make your own delicious **FODMAP**-friendly dip.

4 to 5 red bell peppers (2 pounds/1 kg)

5 ounces (150 g) Danish or regular feta

Juice of 1 lemon

¼ cup (60 ml) extra virgin olive oil

1 teaspoon sea salt

Pinch of red pepper flakes, or to taste

Freshly cracked black pepper, to taste

1. Preheat the oven to 350°F (180°C) and line a baking sheet with parchment paper.
2. Cut the peppers in half and remove the seeds before placing them, skin side up, on the baking sheet. Bake for 30 minutes to 1 hour, depending on how big your peppers are. Their flesh should be softened and their skin blistered.
3. Transfer to a bowl and cover with a kitchen towel to encourage them to sweat as they cool. This makes it easy-peasy to peel them.
4. Peel the peppers and add the flesh to a food processor along with all the other ingredients. Pulse until you achieve your desired dip consistency—I like mine chunky.
5. Taste and adjust for seasoning and flavor, then serve. Store in an airtight container in the fridge for up to 3 days.

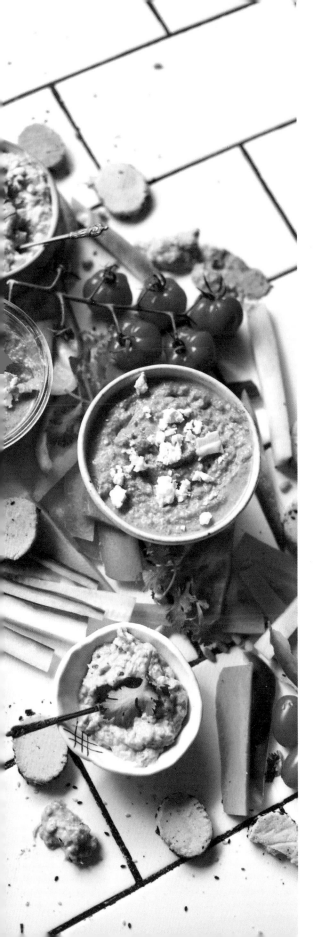

Baba Ghanoush

MAKES ENOUGH
FOR 1 MEDIUM
SERVING BOWL

I initially set about creating this recipe as a substitute for hummus. Turns out there is a name for hummus-y flavors combined with eggplant: baba ghanoush! Serve this with Coconut Flatbreads (page 111), Tempeh Nut Falafels (page 70), or crudités.

1 large eggplant (about 1 pound/500 g), halved lengthwise, flesh scored
Juice of 1 lemon
1 piece (20 g) preserved lemon rind, finely chopped
2 teaspoons preserved lemon brine
2 teaspoons light olive oil
Good pinch of sea salt
Good pinch of cracked black pepper
2½ tablespoons extra virgin olive oil
2½ tablespoons tahini
1 teaspoon ground cumin

1. Preheat the oven to 350°F (180°C). Line a baking sheet with parchment paper and lay the eggplants on it flesh side up.
2. In a small bowl, combine half of the lemon juice and half of the preserved lemon with the lemon brine and light olive oil. Add the salt and pepper. Liberally coat the eggplants with this mixture.
3. Roast for 30 minutes, then gently flip the eggplants over and roast for another 20 minutes, or until soft. Remove from the oven and cool completely.
4. Spoon the eggplant flesh into a food processor and discard the skins. Add the remaining ingredients, including the remaining lemon juice and preserved lemon, and process until smooth. Serve, or store in the fridge for up to 3 days.

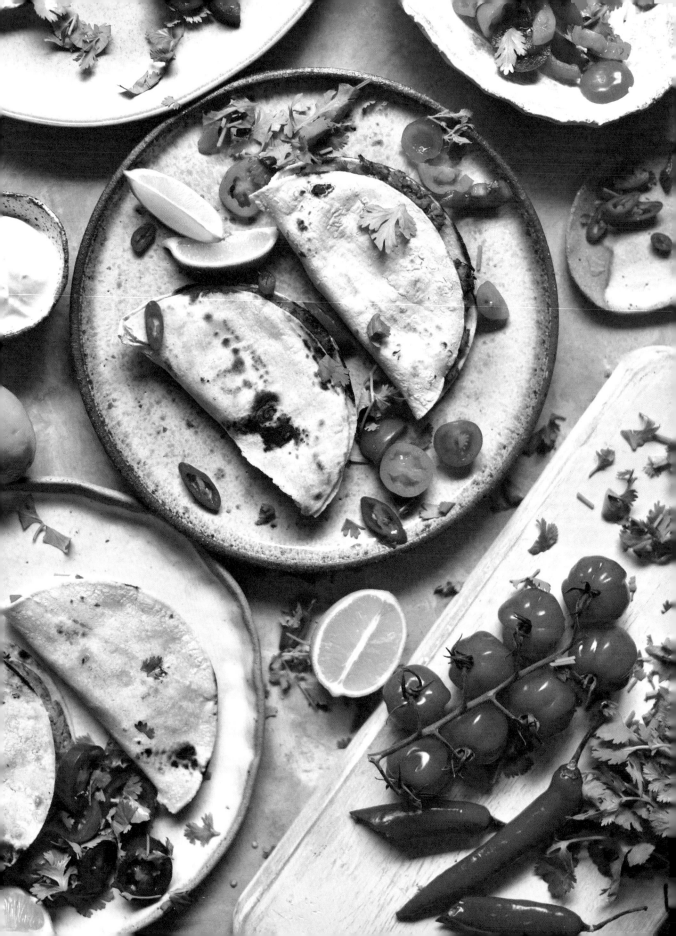

"Refried Bean" Quesadillas

SERVES
4 TO 5

One food I've struggled to relinquish from my previous FODMAP-ignorant life is canned refried beans (this is a no-judgment zone, remember?). They were an integral part of taco night in our predominantly vegetarian household. These days, the thought of eating beans makes my digestive system shudder, so this tempeh version makes a great stand-in. Keep in mind that tempeh is high in oligos at 7 ounces (220 g) per serving, so maybe just don't eat six out of the ten quesadillas. You can use coconut yogurt instead of sour cream and vegan cheese instead of cheddar if you'd like to keep these vegan.

Tempeh paste

14 ounces (400 g) tempeh
1 bunch cilantro, stems included
  (reserve a small handful for
  the salsa)
1 tablespoon vegetable oil
1 tablespoon ground cumin
1 tablespoon smoked paprika
2 teaspoons ground coriander
2 teaspoons gluten-free tamari
Zest of ½ lime
Juice of 1 lime
1 jalapeño, roughly chopped
Red pepper flakes, to taste
Sea salt, to taste
Cracked black pepper, to taste

Salsa

1 pint (10 ounces/300 g) cherry
  tomatoes
Pinch of lime zest (optional)
Juice of ½ lime
Pinch of sea salt

Quesadillas

10 gluten-free tortillas
1⅓ cups (150 g) freshly grated
  good-quality cheddar
⅔ cup (150 g) sour cream
  (1 tablespoon per quesadilla)
Neutral oil spray
Lime wedges, to serve

1. Preheat the oven to 300°F (150°C).
2. **To make the tempeh paste,** combine all the ingredients with ½ cup (120 ml) water in a food processor and blend until you have a paste the consistency of refried beans. (If you have an older blender, you may need to chop your cilantro quite well beforehand.) Set aside.
3. **To make the salsa,** chop the cherry tomatoes and the reserved cilantro. Transfer to a bowl with the lime zest, if you want extra zing, lime juice, and salt. Set aside.
4. **To make the quesadillas,** warm the tortillas by wrapping them in foil and placing them in the oven for a few minutes.
5. Spread an even amount of tempeh paste on one half of each tortilla, leaving room to fold them in half. Top the tempeh paste with the salsa, cheese, and sour cream, then gently fold the tortillas and press down to fasten them. The tortillas might crack a little, and that's OK. (Don't we all, really?)
6. Heat a griddle pan over medium heat and, with a spray of oil, lightly brown each tortilla on both sides before transferring to the oven to keep warm. A bit of color is ideal.
7. Serve with any remaining salsa, additional sour cream, and some lime wedges.

Smoky Popcorn and Salted Caramel Popcorn

MAKES A SMALL BOWL OF POPCORN

Nothing says "I won't be getting off the couch tonight" quite like whipping up a batch of popcorn. To help you nail all your Netflix binge goals I've included a sweet *and* a savory variety. Both are super easy to whip up—ensuring you can focus all your energy on the marathon at hand.

3 teaspoons vegetable oil
¼ cup (50 g) unpopped popcorn

Smoky popcorn
1 tablespoon maple syrup
1 teaspoon smoked paprika
1 teaspoon pumpkin pie spice
1 teaspoon salt
1½ tablespoons (25 g) butter

Salted caramel popcorn
¼ cup (30 g) light brown or
   coconut sugar
¼ cup (30 g) coconut milk (make
   sure it doesn't contain inulin)
Dash of vanilla bean paste or
   extract
Sea salt, to taste
Small handful of banana chips,
   roughly chopped (optional)

1. **To make the popcorn,** heat the oil in a medium saucepan over medium-high heat. Add the popcorn kernels and, shaking regularly, allow the kernels to pop. Keep checking on the popcorn to make sure you don't burn it—there are few things as disheartening as a burnt batch of popcorn. Remove from the heat and set aside.

2. **To make the smoky popcorn,** mix the maple syrup, spices, and salt in a small bowl to make a paste. Stir the butter into the popcorn, followed by the spice paste.

3. **To make the salted caramel popcorn,** cook the sugar and coconut milk with the vanilla in a saucepan for 3 to 5 minutes, until it becomes sauce-like. Add the salt and pour the caramel over the popcorn while it is still in the pan. Stir the mixture gently before serving and add some banana chips, if you like.

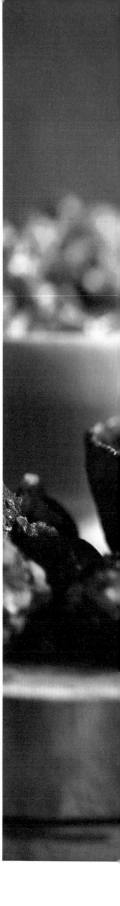

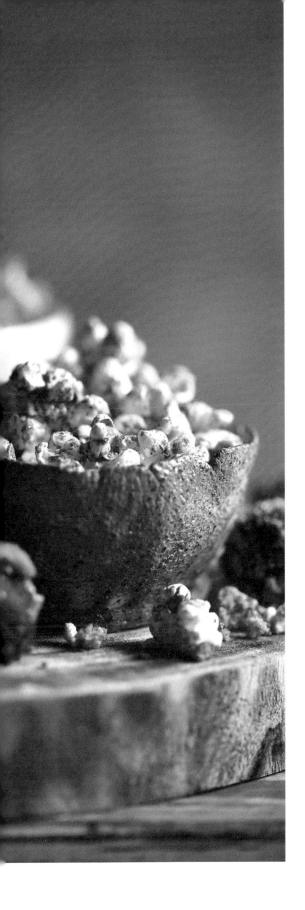

Chocolate and Peanut Butter Truffles

Not one to miss out on a treat whose primary ingredient is peanut butter, I initially set about creating these as a fructose-friendly "bliss ball." As it turns out, they work equally as well (if not better) as a truffle. They are free of dairy, gluten, grains, refined sugars, and, most importantly, damn dates. You can roll them in your choice of toppings; I use crushed freeze-dried berries, but shredded coconut, cocoa powder, or cacao nibs also work well.

½ cup (140 g) natural peanut butter
1 tablespoon pure maple syrup
1 teaspoon butter or coconut butter
2½ tablespoons cocoa powder
1 tablespoon coconut sugar
Sprinkle of fine salt
Crushed freeze-dried raspberries or shredded coconut, to serve (optional)

1. Stir together the peanut butter, maple syrup, and butter in a medium bowl. The trick is to continue stirring long after the ingredients have combined—the longer you stir, the thicker and tougher it gets. Stir for at least 2 minutes.
2. Add the cocoa, coconut sugar, and salt and stir to combine. Use your hands to shape ten or so small truffles from the mixture. Roll them in the raspberries, if using.
3. Store in an airtight container in the fridge, and eat within 3 to 5 days.

Christmas Pudding

"It tastes better than normal Christmas pudding"—a review from a friend who would definitely tell me if it didn't. This magical Christmas pudding is completely fruit-free—it uses candied squash instead. It's also gluten- and grain-free, so you can be dietary-niche Santa on Christmas Day. Serve this with lactose-free custard or ice cream and some berries.

1 recipe "Fruit" Mince (page 180)
3 extra-large eggs
1 cup (100 g) almond meal
¾ cup (75 g) tapioca flour
5 tablespoons (75 g) butter, melted and cooled
¼ cup (30 g) dark brown sugar, not packed
2½ tablespoons Campari
1 teaspoon ground cinnamon
1 teaspoon ground nutmeg
½ teaspoon ground clove
Pinch of fine salt

1. Fill the bottom of a large soup pot with water. Place something waterproof and crack-proof on the bottom so that the pudding is elevated just above the water. I used an inverted steel pie pan.

2. Grease a pudding bowl or basin liberally. (A similar heatproof bowl will work in a pinch, but if the pudding is flatter, the cook time may be shorter.) You can line the circular base of the pudding bowl as an insurance policy, if you like.

3. Mix together all the ingredients in a large bowl and transfer to the pudding bowl. You can place a piece of parchment paper on the bottom of the pudding, too—this will prevent any rogue water from getting in and will also result in a smooth base.

4. Layer two pieces of foil over the pudding and secure tightly with string. Place the pudding on the little island you've created and pop the lid on. Turn the heat to medium-low and cook for 2 hours.

5. Open the pudding carefully so that you can continue to cook if necessary, but also so you don't get a steam burn. If there is a bit of squishiness when you press the center, cook in additional 15-minute increments until it feels completely firm.

6. Allow to cool a little before gently running a knife around the edge (if necessary) and inverting onto a plate to serve.

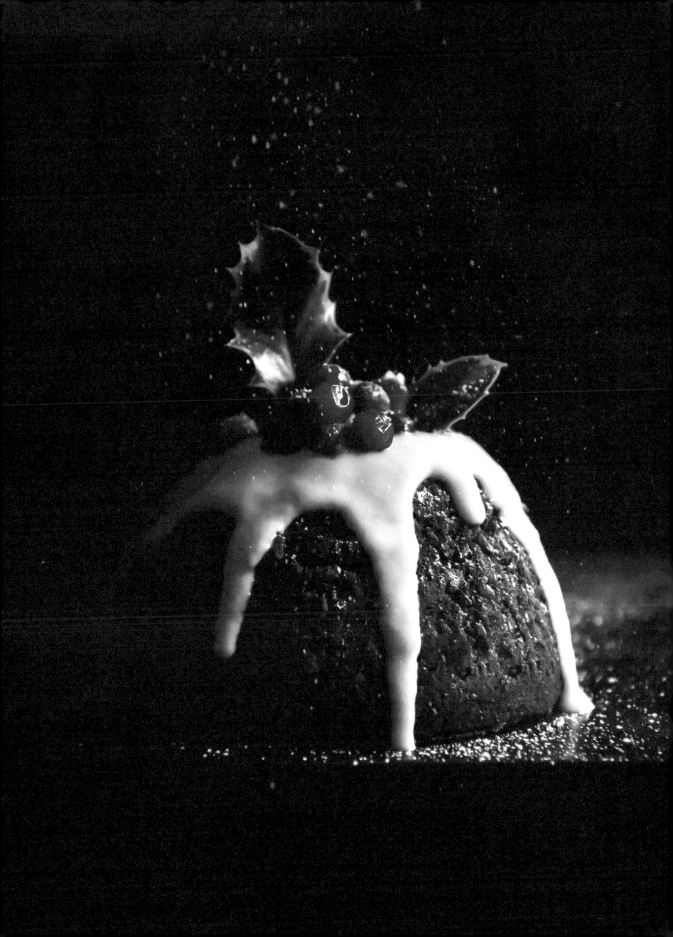

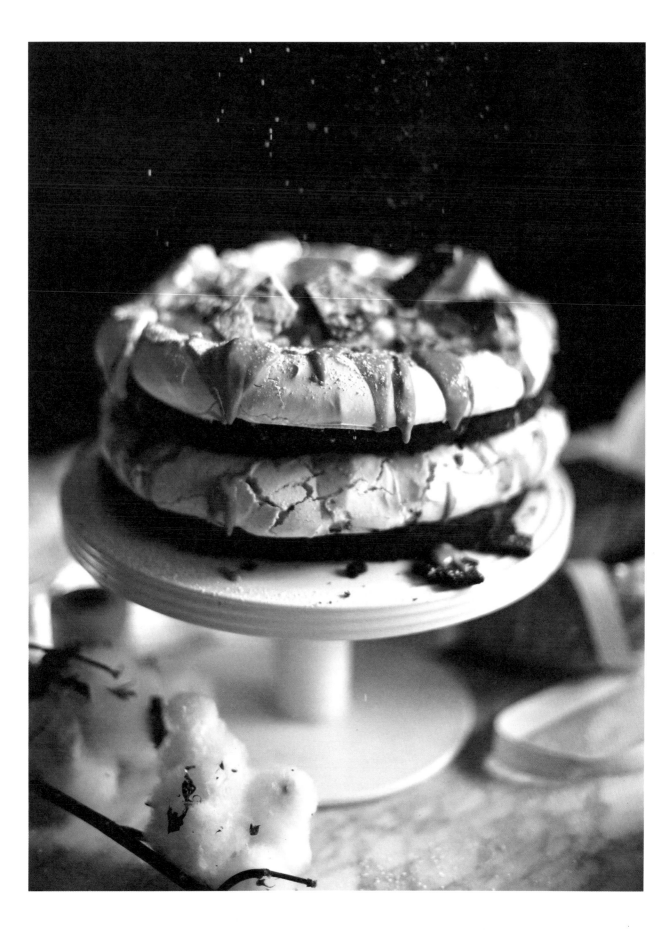

Chocolate and Meringue Celebration Layer Cake

SERVES **10 TO 12**

So you need a cake that says, "I made an otherworldly amount of effort and you should fawn over me and my culinary abilities?" Say no more, fam. I got you.

Olive oil spray

1 recipe Meringue (page 156), not spread out or baked

1 Grain-Free Chocolate Cake (page 152)

½ cup (140 g) natural peanut butter (see Note)

¼ cup (40 g) freshly toasted peanuts

Chocolate shards and confectioners' sugar, to decorate

1. Preheat the oven to 400°F (200°C). Spray two baking sheets with olive oil and lay a sheet of parchment paper on top of each (the oil will stop the paper from sliding around when you spread the meringue).

2. Divide the uncooked meringue in half and, using a spatula, spread each portion onto the center of a baking sheet in a disk measuring roughly 9 inches (23 cm).

3. Pop in the oven and immediately turn the heat down to 250°F (120°C). Cook for 45 minutes to 1 hour, intermittently checking that the meringues haven't gone brown. The cooking time may vary depending on your oven, so keep a close eye on them. They should be pale and firm outside but soft inside. Switch the oven off, leaving the meringues in there to cool completely with the oven door ajar.

4. Carefully halve the chocolate cake horizontally and place the bottom of the cake on your serving platter of choice.

5. Lightly spread half of the peanut butter over the cake base and then stick the first meringue on top.

6. Stack the other cake half on top, spread on the remaining peanut butter (reserving some to top, if desired), and follow with the last meringue. Top with the peanuts, any reserved peanut butter, some chocolate shards, and a dusting of sugar.

Note: For peanut allergy sufferers, you can substitute the peanut butter and toasted peanuts with another nut of your choosing. Just keep in mind that the chocolate cake contains almond meal, so these substitutions alone won't be appropriate for a broad nut allergy.

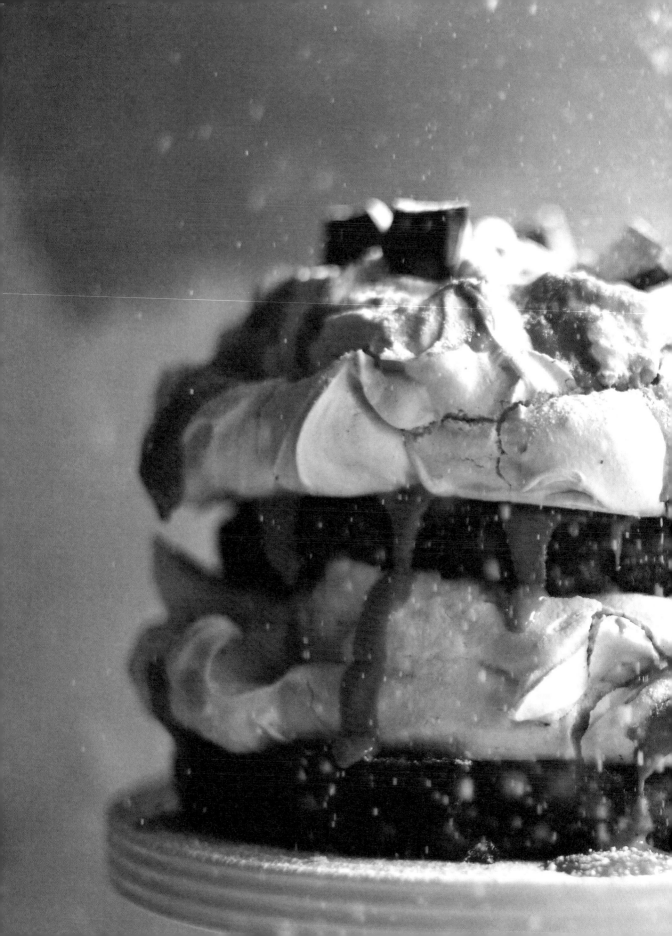

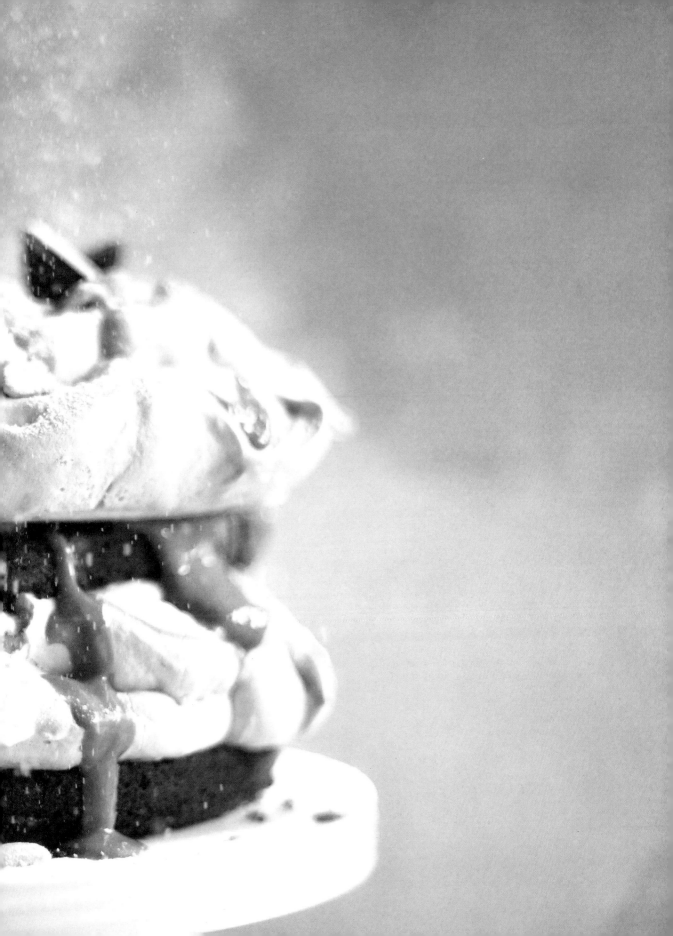

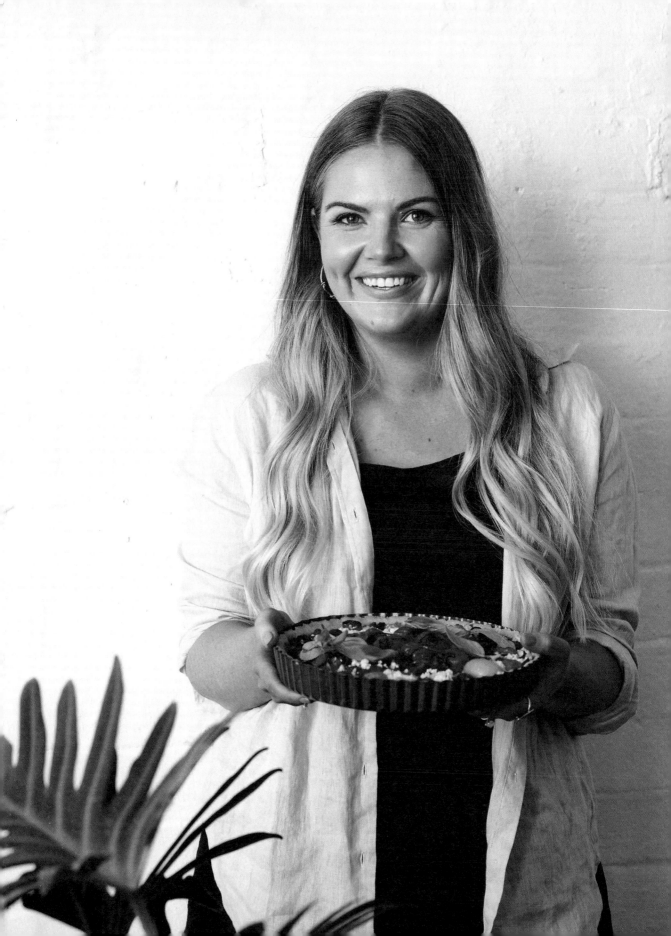

Acknowledgments

To my mum, for being the backbone of this whole book, without whom I would have been an inconsolable, directionless, anxiety-ridden mess for nine months. For all the trips to the shops (five times in one day was our record, I think?), for the moral support, and for the endless and occasionally unwelcome honesty, I probably can't thank you enough. I am quite confident I couldn't have achieved this without you.

To my dad, for consuming all my terrible recipe tests with enthusiasm and appreciation. For all the grammar corrections, the Instagram likes (he has three identical personal accounts from which he religiously likes all my Instagram posts)—I probably couldn't have gained notoriety without your 3x support.

To my sister, who'd not only be outraged if I weren't to include her, but who has self-proclaimed herself the Georgeats hand model, despite living a world away in London. Thanks for all that quality hand modeling once every two years, Sis.

To my friends and family, who have accepted, nay, encouraged, me to crouch over food on the floor for a living, since day one. For allowing me to be absent for a whole year, for motivating me, and for showing up, whether that be to hand model (see the fine specimens in the group shots for but one example), to taste test, or just to pat me on the back and provide the wine while I fall in an anxious heap. You're A+. Special mention

to Liana, whose weekly volunteer hand modeling was instrumental in paying my rent for a solid two years.

To my Instagram followers (who am I?)—you are the reason I'm currently writing these acknowledgments. Not to be a giant millennial cliché, but when I first started secretly photographing and uploading my food for the 'gram, I never in a million years dreamed that it would become what it has today. I have you all to thank. Without your support, your encouragement, your comments—my life would have taken an entirely different trajectory. I'm so utterly #blessed and grateful that I could cry some ugly tears into my laptop. Please picture this while you're cooking something from the book.

To Olivia and the team at The Experiment Publishing—thank you for everything. Your professionalism, encouragement, openness, and patience have been incredibly refreshing, and I'm so humbled to have the opportunity to publish with you in the American market. You've been an absolute dream to work with and I can't wait to see where our partnership goes!

Finally, thank you for buying the book (or skimming it covertly at the bookstore)—see above reference to overused hashtags and ugly crying.

Index

NOTE: Page numbers in *italics* indicate a photograph.

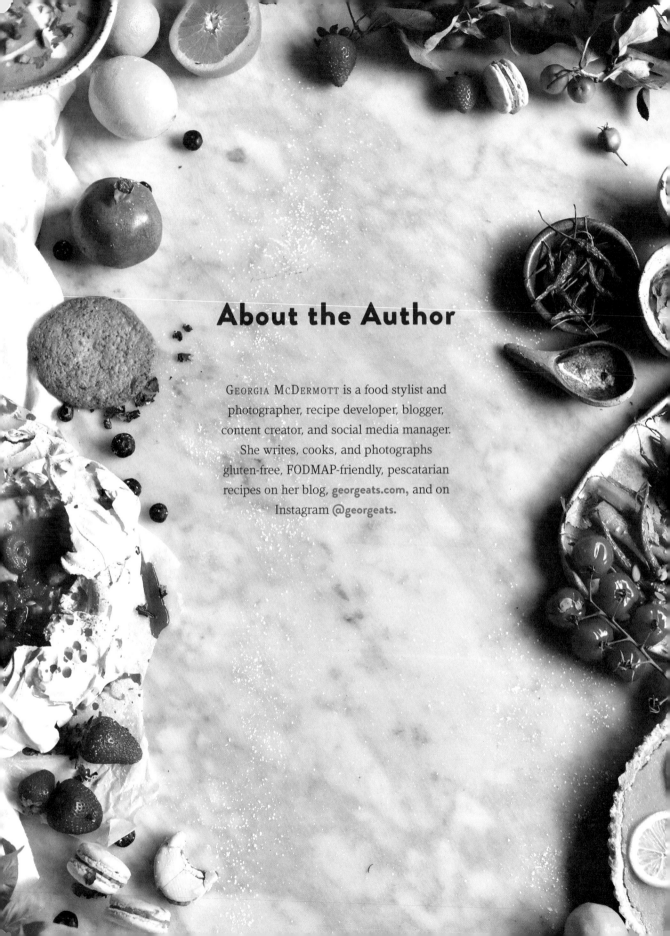

About the Author

GEORGIA MCDERMOTT is a food stylist and
photographer, recipe developer, blogger,
content creator, and social media manager.
She writes, cooks, and photographs
gluten-free, FODMAP-friendly, pescatarian
recipes on her blog, **georgeats.com,** and on
Instagram @georgeats.